PHYSICAL ACTIVITY
AND AGING

American Academy
of Physical Education Papers
No. 22

PHYSICAL ACTIVITY AND AGING

American Academy
of Physical Education Papers
No. 22

Sixtieth Annual Meeting
Kansas City, Missouri
April 5–6, 1988

Published by Human Kinetics Books
for the American Academy of Physical Education

Editors
Waneen W. Spirduso
Helen M. Eckert

Academy Seal designed by
R. Tait McKenzie

Managing Editor: Peg Goyette
Typesetter: Angela Snyder

ISBN 0-87322-220-2
ISSN 0741-4633

Library of Congress Cataloging-in-Publication Data

American Academy of Physical Education. Meeting
   (60th : 1988 : Kansas City, Mo.)
   Physical activity and aging.

   (American Academy of Physical Education Papers ; no. 22)
   Includes bibliographies.
   1. Physical education for the aged--Congresses.
2. Exercise for the aged--Congresses. 3. Aging--
Congresses. I. Title. II. Series: American
Academy of Physical Education. Meeting. Academy papers ; no. 22.
GV447.A48   1988   613.7'0240565   88-26597
ISBN 0-87322-220-2

Printed in the United States of America   6 5 4

Human Kinetics
P.O. Box 5076, Champaign, IL 61825-5076
1-800-747-4457

Canada: Human Kinetics, Box 24040, Windsor, ON N8Y 4Y9
1-800-465-7301 (in Canada only)

Europe: Human Kinetics, P.O. Box IW14, Leeds LS16 6TR, England
0532-781708

Australia: Human Kinetics, P.O. Box 80, Kingswood 5062, South Australia
618-374-0433

New Zealand: Human Kinetics, P.O. Box 105-231, Auckland 1
(09) 309-2259

CONTENTS

88362

Physical Activity and Aging: Introduction

Waneen W. Spirduso
University of Texas at Austin

It is no secret that America is aging. The over-65 age group is the fastest grow-ing age group in our society. The most dramatic way to describe the demograph-ic age changes is to compare the number of individuals who were over 65 in 1900 with the number who will be over 65 in the year 2000 (Figure 1). In 1900 only 4% of the population, or 123,000 people, were 65 or older. In 2000 it is project-ed that 32 million people, or 15–20%, will be in that age category. While the percent of our population that this group represents will increase only about three or four times, the absolute number of individuals this age will be staggering. "In 1983 there were more people over the age of 65 than there were teenagers, and (because of the Baby Boom growing old) that condition remains a constant for as long as any of us live. America will simply not be a nation of young in our lifetime. The only growth area in education will be adult and continuing educa-tion, with growth in elementary schools in certain regions" (Hodgkinson, 1985).

Even more astounding is the increase in individuals who are 85 or older. In each decade since 1940 the population of these individuals has increased by greater than 50%. In 1960 less than a million people were older than 85. By 1980, 2.2 million individuals were that age. It is projected that by the year 2050 there will be 16 million individuals 85 years of age or older, and they will comprise 5% of the population.

We've come a long way in our medical and health quest to postpone death. Better housing and sanitation, less crowding, cleaner and more federal and state regulated food supplies, and improved nutrition have contributed to increased longevity. Antibiotics, vaccines, and blood pressure control techniques have reduced the number of premature deaths. Miraculous surgical procedures that have become commonplace have extended the lives of millions. Health educa-tion has been extremely effective in reducing smoking, improving dietary habits, and controlling stress. Adult exercise programs have helped to make people more physically fit.

The result of our unprecedented success in health promotion and maintenance is that more and more individuals are approaching the upper limits of the human life span. Maximum longevity in the human species is considered to be about 115 years. The human life span is about 85 ± 5 years. The average life expec-tancy, the age that individuals can expect to reach, is about 77 for females and 71 for males. Obviously, individuals who achieve the full human life span add

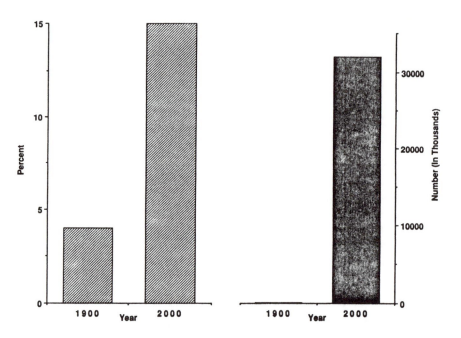

20th Century Over Age 65 Data

Figure 1 — Increases in individuals over the age of 65 shown as percentage of the population (left) and in absolute numbers (right). The numbers of individuals are in thousands; units shown on the right represent 10, 20, and 30 million individuals. Note that in 1900 the absolute number of individuals over the age of 65 was only 125,000, or just a little over 1/10th of 1 million people.

more years to their lives. But the question of major importance to both the individual and society is, "Is increasing the age at death adding quality years to life or is it increasing the period of disease state and morbidity that precedes death?" Roy Walford suggested in his Kleemeir Award presentation that individuals should probably be thinking about achieving an average *health expectancy* rather than an average *life expectancy* (1980).

The duration of morbidity, that is, a period of time preceding death in which an individual is permanently ill or infirm, has awesome social, personal, and medical implications. A long period of morbidity can result in individual suffering, personal financial ruin, and societal bankruptcy due to health service costs. If the period of morbidity can be compressed, as suggested by Fries' Compression of Morbidity model (1980, 1984; Myers & Manton, 1984), then the additional years would extend the collective knowledge, wisdom, and judgment of the society. Bonus years at the end of a well-planned and healthful life would provide the individual with an enriched period of time in which to reflect over a mosaic of cherished memories as well as to synthesize and culminate projects so that life goals are fulfilled.

Failure to compress the period of morbidity, as well as the period of chronic age-related illness that institutionalizes people and precedes morbidity, would be a social and economic disaster. The health care costs of those over 65 years of age, which are triple those of younger individuals, represented 29% of the total health care costs in 1980 in the United States. Three percent of the gross national product, or $100 billion, is spent on the health of those over 65. One third of that $100 billion is spent on the last year of life in the elderly population. In 1982 only 5% of the elderly population was institutionalized, yet that 5% cost $25 billion, and it is predicted that these costs will be $75 billion in 1990 for this group alone.

The compression of morbidity and premorbidity dysfunctional states will require preventive approaches to premature chronic disease, changes in social expectations, and positive programs for reducing the burden of illness. Preventive approaches certainly will include physical activity as an integral component. Evidence now supports the proposition that more than half of the decline of physical capacity in older individuals is due to boredom, inactivity, and expected infirmity. Professionals as well as the general public are becoming aware that maintaining physical activity in the life of a septuagenarian or octogenarian is crucial to a successful aging. But this awareness, although dawning in a growing group of devotees, is relatively new. Although we predict that systematic and intelligent physical activity programs have great potential to enhance health in the aging, we do not yet know the ceiling of benefit, the rate at which it can be attained, or the cost of physical activity to the individual.

In this issue of *The Academy Papers,* authorities in the field of physical activity address the major issues associated with the contributions of health, fitness, and motor skill to successful aging. The extent, nature, and pattern by which muscular coordination and strength decline, with special reference to problems of balance, will be discussed. What types of muscular weakness are seen? Do muscle groups lose strength differentially? Can strength training programs prevent falling? Can strength training programs begun late in life have beneficial effects? How late in life can they be started? Does the loss of strength affect coordination? What types of coordination are affected? Can coordination lost through disuse be regained with practice?

Other questions that are addressed are the effects of chronic physical activity on the cardiovascular system. How does exercise affect hypertension? Many older individuals are adhering to prescribed medication protocols. Given that drug clearance profiles of older individuals cannot be predicted according to those of young individuals, how does exercise interact with medication programs prescribed for age-related problems such as hypothyroidism and hypertension? Does exercise help prevent osteoporosis in older women?

Systematic physical activity appears also to have benefits that go beyond the enhancement and maintenance of physical capacity. Many investigators have suggested that chronic physical activity has beneficial effects on the central nervous system, so that mental functioning, as expressed by psychomotor behaviors, and neuropsychological functioning, as shown in some types of neuropsychological diagnostic tests, are maintained in healthy and physically fit individuals. But how much physical activity is necessary to see these benefits, and how early in life must the physical activity be initiated? Are these benefits related to the physiological change that occurs as a result of exercise programs, or are they fringe benefits of a healthy, vigorous, and optimistic personality? Personality characteristics tend to be relatively stable across life, so that the ways of facing the world tend to be lifelong patterns. A lifelong pattern of optimism, self-confidence, and stimulus-seeking behavior might very well be more effective in maintaining health than a pattern of forced exercise. James Birren, who for years directed the famous Andrus Gerontology Center at the University of Southern California, once said, "It used to be that physiologists would say, 'Do you really mean that the way we think influences our health?' Then I couldn't be sure. Today I say absolutely. . . . We now realize that the way we feel, think, and behave influences how long we're going to live" (personal communication).

Health and exercise effects on physical capacities can readily be measured, but other psychological and social benefits, not so easily measured, probably also accrue to the active individual. What is the role of physical fitness in the psychological health of an individual? How does it contribute to mental health, stress reduction, attitudes, and the feelings of life satisfaction that people have? How does the self-concept, self-esteem, and body image of physically fit and healthy older individuals compare to those of the infirm or chronically ill? Can exercise reduce psychological depression, a common problem in the aged? And what of the feelings that individuals have about the aesthetics of their body and its ability to move? How do they deal with a deteriorating physical structure, which betrays them in their locomotor and manipulative skills and has for so long been a large part of how others view them as a person? To what extent can physical fitness maintain individuals' views about their appearance and ease of movement as the body ages?

The following chapters will show that, on the whole, the literature supports the notion that although there are risks and costs associated with a lifestyle of physical activity, the benefits outweigh the costs. Physical activity is prescribed for individuals at all ages, but parameters of an ideal exercise and health program for individuals of different ages have not yet been clarified. Exercise prescriptions for the elderly continue to be largely guesswork for those in an exercise leadership capacity. Discussed in one chapter are factors affecting appropriate exercise prescriptions for the elderly, while another chapter will address the special problem of adherence to exercise programs. It is often difficult for older adults to adhere to exercise regimens. The change in appearance, the loss of physical capacity, the loss of friends with whom to exercise, and the lack of transportation all serve to discourage the very old from participating in organized physical activity programs.

A lifestyle of physical activity appears to be an extremely important component in the preventive health model that must supplant the medical treatment model of today if this country is to remain economically, psychologically, and socially robust, healthy, and competitive. It is a major responsibility of the physical education profession and related health fields to clarify the benefits, risks, and specific parameters of physical activity, to publicize them, and to develop physical activity prescriptions and programs that are appropriate for individuals of all ages. It is toward the clarification of benefits, risks, and parameters of physical activity that the American Academy of Physical Education turns its attention in this volume.

REFERENCES

FRIES, J.F. (1980). Aging, natural death, and the compression of morbidity. *The New England Journal of Medicine, 303,* 130-135.

FRIES, J.F. (1984). The compression of morbidity: Miscellaneous comments about a theme. *The Gerontologist, 24,* 354-359.

HODGKINSON, H.L. (1985). *All one system: Demographics of education. Kindergarten through graduate school* (pp. 1-18). Washington, DC: Institute for Educational Leadership.

MYERS, G.C., & Manton, K.G. (1984). Compression of mortality: Myth or reality? *The Gerontologist, 24,* 346-353.

WALFORD, R. (1980, November). The Kleemeir Award Presentation, Gerontological Society of America, San Diego.

Psychomotor Decline With Age

George E. Stelmach and Noreen L. Goggin
University of Wisconsin at Madison

With advancing age comes some slowing in performance. This article will review age-related declines in the preparation and execution of movements. While a review of changes in the control of human movements is methodologically complex due to the contributions of physiological, behavioral, and health factors, an important question that needs to be examined is whether the aging nervous system can integrate sensory information to prepare and/or correct motor system output (Ochs, Newberry, Lenhardt, & Harkins, 1985). Often the motor system is unable to "react" to sensory information fast enough to produce a response. This difficulty has a variety of implications for everyday life of older individuals: daily living tasks may be hampered (Salthouse, 1985), slowness of behavior with increased age may prevent success for older workers in industrial settings (Welford, 1977), and, more important, there is a 33% chance that an older person will suffer a damaging fall by the time he or she reaches 80 years of age (Stelmach & Worringham, 1985). The present review will consider the psychomotor changes that occur with increased age. Specifically, data will be presented that document the slowness of response initiation—reaction time (RT), response execution deficits—movement time (MT), and changes in the control aspects of movement.

SLOWNESS OF RESPONSE INITIATION (RT)

Central mechanisms have been implicated in the slowing of performance with age. Welford (1984b) argues that psychomotor slowing is the result of central or *cognitive* mechanisms rather than peripheral or reflex mechanisms. Thus, RT techniques are used to estimate the time of various cognitive processes. Simple and choice RT tasks have shown that as one ages, central mechanisms are impaired (see Table 1) and consequently a slowing of response initiation is seen (Cerella, 1985; Gottsdanker, 1982). Age deficits are also seen in manipulations of task complexity (Jordan & Rabbitt, 1977), preparation of movement (Gottsdanker, 1980b), changes in stimulus–response compatibility (Rabbitt, 1979), speed–accuracy relationships (Salthouse, 1979), and in postural control (Mankovskii, Mints, & Lysenyuk, 1980; Woollacott, Shumway-Cook, & Nashner, 1982). However, it is not clear whether there are generalized deficits in central mechanisms or whether aging has specific effects upon one aspect of cognitive–motor processing in particular.

Table 1

Reaction Time and Movement Time (MS) Deficits With Age

Criterion measure	Condition	Young	Older	% Difference
Clarkson (1978)				
Total RT	Simple	216	261	21
	choice	247	307	24
Premotor time	Simple	129	162	26
	choice	151	194	28
Motor time	Simple	87	98	13
	choice	96	112	17
MT	Simple	124	164	32
	choice	130	170	31
Jordan & Rabbitt (1977)				
Total RT	Simple	531	582	10
	choice	977	1294	32
Larish & Stelmach (1982)				
Total RT	Probability			
	80%	250	325	30
	50%	270	360	33
	20%	280	380	36
MT	Probability			
	80%	185	225	22
	50%	193	215	11
	20%	187	230	23
Szafran (1951)				
Total RT	Choice	860	1370	59
MT	Choice	1180	1220	3
Weiss (1965)				
Total RT	Simple	174	228	31
Premotor time	Simple	109	153	40
Motor time	Simple	65	75	15

Although a variety of RT techniques have implicated central processing deficits, it is difficult to rule out peripheral problems. Salthouse (1985) has proposed several hypotheses that describe and account for the slowness of reaction time. One hypothesis deals with the slowness of transmitting information between the central nervous system and the peripheral output system, which he terms "input or output rate." The changes in the peripheral system that occur with advanced age are thought to produce the delays in the transmission of information. These peripheral factors may contribute to the slowing, but certainly are not responsible for all slowing observed in older individuals. Weiss (1965) and Clarkson (1978) fractionated RT into two components to determine whether central or peripheral factors were responsible for the slowing of RT that comes with age. These studies suggest that peripheral processes remain intact with increasing age and the RT deficits in older adults are due to central processing deficits.

Weiss (1965) examined the effect of set, motivation, and age on the performance of a simple RT task. The first component of the RT is the premotor time (PMT) and reflects the time necessary for signal reception by the sense organs, the processing of the signal, and impulses sent from the brain to the corresponding muscles. The other component is motor time, which is the time from onset of EMG signals in the muscle to the initiation of the desired response. Weiss found that the predominant differences between old and young subjects were in the PMT component. Clarkson (1978) studied knee extension response time in active and inactive young and older adults. She found that the PMT component increased with age and was higher in inactive older adults. Thus, using the fractionization technique provides additional information on the locus of the RT deficits.

A second plausible explanation proposed by Salthouse (1985) for aging deficits in speed of processing deals with central mechanism deficits called "hardware differences," which are internal mechanisms responsible for the operation of the cognitive–motor system. A major theory attributing slowness to hardware differences in older adults is the neural noise hypothesis proposed by Welford (1981, 1982, 1984a). Welford proposes that the signal-to-noise ratio in older adults is much smaller than the ratio in young people. This could be due to weaker signals, increased noise, or a combination of the two (Welford, 1981), which causes RT to increase because of central transmission deficits.

A final explanation proposed by Salthouse (1985) which localizes deficits to one particular aspect of the information processing system is termed "software differences." These include the sequences of control processes, strategy differences, poor preparation, task complexity, and speed–accuracy trade-offs, which all seem to be affected by age.

While there is evidence to support the explanations proposed by Salthouse (1985), there are data that suggest that older adults shift control from open- to closed-loop mechanisms. Rabbitt (1982) has discussed control strategies as being either *predictive*, that is, having the ability to initiate complex motor patterns in anticipation of changes that are about to occur, or *reactive,* using feedback to initiate complex patterns of corrective movements. He feels that the young have the ability to use either predictive or reactive control when necessary. However, older adults gradually lose the option of predictive control and have to maintain reactive control as best they can. This loss of predictive control can also be seen in postural control in a feedforward mechanism known as a preparatory postural adjustment, which occurs prior to the onset of voluntary movement. Young subjects, prior to the initiation of a voluntary movement, perform opposing preparatory stural responses so that voluntary movement does not move the body's center of gravity beyond the base of support (Bouisett & Zattara, 1981). These adjustments reduce instability caused by the upcoming voluntary movement. Mankovskii et al. (1980) found that older persons made minimum postural adjustments when performing voluntary responses; consequently, this poor coordination was accompanied by increased postural instability. It has been hypothesized that the inability to make postural adjustments may cause instability to occur during rapid voluntary movements while standing (Stelmach & Worringham, 1985).

Although it is quite clear that RT increases with advancing age, some research suggests that such RT increases can be minimized or prevented. Spirduso (1982) has shown that physical exercise alters the rate of decline in some physiological and cognitive functions. That is, physically trained older adults have much faster RTs than age-matched untrained older adults. She has indicated that many of the physiological and cognitive changes that accompany normal aging can be minimized by engaging in physical exercise. It has also been found that practice is much more beneficial for older adults (Spirduso, 1982), and RTs of older adults have been shown to decline with extended practice (Salthouse, 1985). Finally, when older adults are allowed to make vocal responses rather than manual responses, the RT differences between young and older adults are not as dramatic (Salthouse, 1985; Salthouse & Somberg, 1982). Although these areas of exercise, practice, and vocal responses appear to cause exceptions to the slowing seen with advanced age, the RT differences between the young and the old cannot be completely eliminated.

POSSIBLE CAUSES FOR SLOWNESS
OF RESPONSE INITIATION (RT)

Given that psychomotor slowing can in part be attributed to central processes, techniques are required to establish which cognitive processes are impaired. For example, manipulating task parameters or providing advance information may help determine the causes of slowing in older adults.

Studies conducted by Gottsdanker (1980a, 1980b) and those performed in our laboratory have provided advance precue information. In addition, manipulation of task parameters has been used to indicate that more complicated movements require more preparation. Gottsdanker (1980a), for example, used a simple RT task to determine the effect of age on advanced preparation: As more information was provided in advance, RTs were postulated to decrease. He found an age difference when movement preparation was manipulated, and concluded that only when preparation was easy were RT differences small between the young and the old subjects. In addition, Gottsdanker (1980b) suggested that older adults have difficulty in preparing and maintaining that movement preparation.

Stelmach, Goggin, and Garcia-Colera (1987) used a response precueing paradigm to determine whether movement planning processes were responsible for slower response initiation times in older individuals. Three groups of subjects (young, middle aged, and older adults) received either no, partial, or complete information about the parameters of arm, direction, and extent prior to the imperative response signal. They hypothesized that older adults would take more time to specify movement dimensions. The results clearly indicated that the older adults had slower RTs and information transmission rates and made more errors. Older adults were able to use advance precue information to prepare the upcoming movement, but their specification times for arm (78 ms for older adults vs. 23 ms for younger subjects) direction (77 vs. 34 ms) and extent (60 vs. 18 ms) were much slower than those of the young, and they had disproportionate increases in RT as a function of response uncertainty (see Figure 1). The data show that part of the slowing of RTs in older adults may be due to the increased time necessary to specify a dimension of movement, and to the uncertainty associated with producing a response.

Stelmach, Amrhein, and Goggin (1988a) used movement reprogramming, SRT, and CRT paradigms to examine the preparation and movement restructuring in older adults. In a reprogramming task, the time required to change a pre-

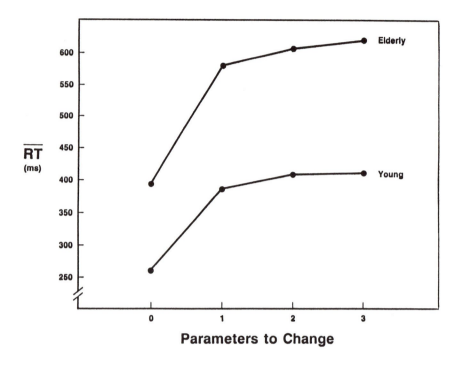

Figure 1 — RT for each age group plotted as a function of uncertainty. *Note*: **Plot is adapted from Stelmach, Goggin, & Garcia-Colera, 1987, "Movement specification time with age,"** *Experimental Aging Research,* **13, 39-46.**

pared movement parameter provides an indication of how long it takes to prepare that parameter. On 75% of the trials in the reprogramming task, the precue specified the target stimulus (valid trials) with respect to the movement parameters of arm and direction. In the remaining trials, the precue incorrectly specified the target stimulus (invalid trials). In addition, a variable interval of 250, 500, 750, or 1000 ms was used between the precue and the response signal to examine the time course of motor plan maintenance and restructuring. The results can be seen in Figure 2 and show that the older adults were slower overall in all tasks and at all precue intervals. The graph also indicates that the best preparation for both groups occurs at the middle intervals of 500 and 750 ms. Across precue intervals, older adults displayed a greater time decrease to restructure a motor plan for direction relative to the other parameter change conditions. This result suggests that there is a loss of preparation for direction with age and it persisted over precue intervals. Thus, it is clear that aging affects motor organization processes differentially at the level of parameter specification.

Larish and Stelmach (1982) and Stelmach, Goggin, and Amrhein (1988) examined conditions in which subjects made movements for which they had advance information that was either valid (programming conditions) or invalid (reprogramming conditions). Thus, it was possible for subjects to prepare the

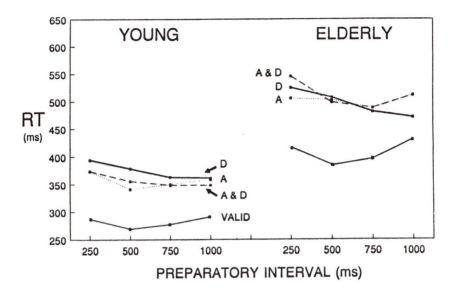

Figure 2 — Effect of age and preparatory interval on valid and invalid trial response latency. *Note:* **Plot is adapted from Stelmach, Amrhein, & Goggin, 1988a, "Maintenance and restructuring of motor preparation with age" (Manuscript in preparation).**

movement prior to the signal, but occasionally it was necessary to restructure the movement at the time of the response signal. The purpose of the experiments was to determine if younger and older adults restructure planned motor responses in a similar fashion. Larish and Stelmach (1982) found that older subjects reacted and moved more slowly than young subjects, but there was no interaction between age and reprogramming conditions. This result indicated that older adults were able to prepare and restructure movements in a similar fashion to young subjects and suggests that the processes responsible for programming and reprogramming are slower but remain intact with advancing age. Stelmach et al. (1988) found slightly different results. The older adults showed proportionally longer RTs overall, which was independent of the requirement to restructure a movement plan. However, this proportionality was not found for the movement parameter of extent: Older adults were disproportionately slower in preparing to make a movement of short extent. These results indicate that with advancing age, the higher level processes (e.g., movement plan restructuring) remain intact, while the structures of some lower level processes (e.g., parameter specification) undergo some change. Therefore, they concluded that older individuals display proportional and disproportional deficits when task parameters are manipulated.

In summary, a portion of the slowness displayed by older adults in response initiation (RT) is caused by their inability to specify movement dimensions and prepare or restructure movement plans. In addition, the RT deficits shown in older adults are contained in central mechanisms, since peripheral processes remain intact with advanced age.

RESPONSE EXECUTION (MT)

The slowness in response preparation in older adults has implications for movement execution. Previous research has found that older adults are slower in response execution (MT) (Welford, 1977, 1982). According to Welford (1984b), the time taken to make a movement reflects the degree of control rather than the time for the muscles to contract and produce the appropriate force. Unlike RT, movement time does not seem to be affected by specification of movement dimensions (Stelmach et al., 1987) or the restructuring of a motor response (Stelmach et al., 1988); thus, MT appears to be unaffected by these mechanisms which are known to cause increases in RT. However, MT is affected by task complexity (Stelmach, Amrhein, & Goggin, 1988b) and target accuracy (Goggin & Christina, 1979; Welford, 1977).

Although earlier studies have not found MT effects for precueing or movement plan restructuring, subsequent studies in our lab have demonstrated some MT effects. An experiment just completed in our lab (Goggin & Stelmach, 1988) assessed age-related differences in kinematic measures of precued movements by manipulating the parameters of direction and extent. Previous precue experiments disregarded the quality of the motor response beyond RT and MT measures. It was hypothesized that kinematic analysis may show "online movement corrections" that occur during movement execution as precued parameter information is varied. It was speculated that there may be less reliance upon preparation and that any unnecessary changes from the prepared movement (due to precueing) may occur during movement execution. Second, it was thought that younger and older adults might show differences in the movement kinematics (i.e., acceleration, deceleration) they produce (Murrell & Entwisle, 1960). Subjects performed short or long movements to the left or the right on a graphics tablet after receiving precue information about the movement.

It was found that older adults had slower RTs and MTs, took longer to reach peak velocity, had smaller peak velocities (see Figure 3), and made more errors. In addition, when direction and extent were both precued all subjects produced higher peak velocities, which indicates that advance information is also helpful during movement execution even though no MT differences were present in precued movements. Older adults weren't able to use the advance information as well as young subjects, since their RTs were slower. An examination of the displacement, velocity, and acceleration traces show that older adults produce movements that are qualitatively different from young subjects.

As was mentioned previously, it has been shown that older adults tend to be slower than young subjects in most tasks that emphasize speeded performance. Part of the slower performance of older adults could be attributed to the notion that they place a greater emphasis on accuracy than young subjects (Welford, 1982). Salthouse (1979) performed several experiments to test this notion and examined RT after manipulating emphasis on speed or accuracy. He found that older adults do place a greater emphasis on accuracy, although the age differences in speed weren't completely accounted for by a speed–accuracy trade-off. Salthouse (1979) suggests that older subjects are more concerned about committing an error than younger subjects, and therefore prefer to operate at a slower movement speed at which errors are less likely. The studies conducted in our laboratory have shown that older adults are slower, but they also produce more

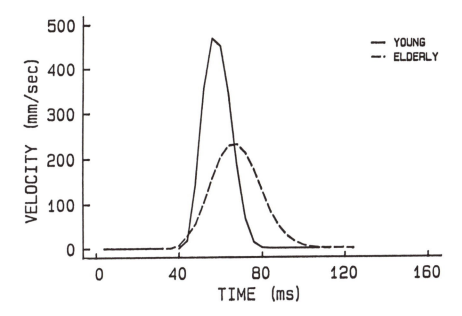

Figure 3 — **Velocity patterns of younger and older subjects.** *Note:* **Plot is adapted from Goggin & Stelmach, 1988, "A kinematic analysis of precued movements in young and elderly subjects" (Manuscript in preparation).**

errors. Thus, it seems unlikely that the emphasis on accuracy by older adults can account completely for the slowness in behavior.

In summary, older individuals are also different from young individuals in response execution. Generally, older adults are slower in their overall MTs and do not show interactions with task manipulations, suggesting MT may be independent of RT. However, it is quite apparent that older adults tend to place more of an emphasis on movement accuracy, which causes MT to increase.

CONTROL ASPECTS OF MOVEMENT

These processes deal with the production of movement and any associated difficulties in the control of movement that older adults might encounter. Research in this area of study indicates that older individuals use different strategies and may emphasize different aspects of movement control than young subjects. For example, older adults tend to be more cautious in their behavior (Salthouse, 1985; Welford, 1984a), show an increased reliance upon vision and visual feedback in the control of movement (Szafran, 1951), demonstrate coordination difficulties (Stelmach et al., 1988b), and have difficulties controlling force (Vrtunski, Patterson, & Hill, 1984).

Welford (1977, 1982, 1984a) has suggested that older people spend more time monitoring their responses, that is, they may inspect the signal for a longer time before responding. He has also suggested that older people are unable to suppress their monitoring, and their frequency of monitoring is higher. He feels that monitoring responses is an aspect of caution in older adult behavior which seems to be an indirect effect of decreasing capacity (Welford, 1981). This cautionary behavior may be an attempt to accumulate more data before acting, as a means of avoiding errors (Welford, 1984a).

Another aspect of control known to be related to movement is the involvement of vision. Szafran (1951) had younger and older adults locate a target with a pointer when they could see their limb, or when only the display could be seen but not the limb. The older adults were slower overall than the young in initiating the movements. Szafran also found that older subjects were much slower than young subjects in locating the target when vision was absent. In addition, older adults made postural adjustments and turned their heads and bodies in an attempt to help relocate the target for which they were aiming. Thus, older adults rely more on visual information than do young people in producing and controlling movement.

The monitoring of responses and the use of vision influence the control of movement in older adults. In performing a movement toward a target, there are two control processes operating: The first is a fast movement concerned with covering the distance, while the second is a slower one "homing in" on the target, which involves visual control and error correction (Warabi, Noda, & Kato, 1986; Welford, 1969). Welford (1969) suggests that the control process dealing with the fast part of the movement declines more with age than do the decisional processes responsible for accuracy of homing on a target. Warabi et al. (1986) used flexion and extension movements of the wrist to follow a target to compare these two phases of control in younger and older adults. Their results indicate that in the first process of moving quickly to the target, peak velocity and amplitude of initial movement remained unchanged with age. However, they found that the duration of the corrective movements, or those responsible for homing on a target, increased with age.

Stelmach et al. (1988b) performed a study to determine if older adults have control problems or deficits in coordinating two hands in a simple motor task. Task complexity was manipulated by using a unimanual task, a symmetric (same extent amplitude) bimanual task and an asymmetric (different extent amplitude) bimanual task. It was hypothesized that older adults should have more difficulty synchronizing asymmetrical movements because of the added dimension of complexity. The results (see Table 2) indicated that the older adults had longer RTs than young subjects across all movement conditions. In addition, all subjects showed an increase in RT across levels of task complexity in movement preparation. Other specific age deficits include poorer preparation of short movements relative to long movements, regardless of task complexity; lessened ability to yoke initiation of bimanual activity; increases in MT with task difficulty; and a poorer ability to compensate for movement initiation asynchrony to terminate movement in a near simultaneous manner. The results indicate that older adults have movement control problems because they display more online movement control and show specific deficits in coordinating two movements.

Other factors known to affect older individuals in producing movements is their ability to control velocity and acceleration and their ability to produce and/or control force. Murrell and Entwisle (1960) examined simple movement patterns

Table 2

Mean Response Initiation (RT) and Mean Response Execution Latency (MT)

Extent	Young		Elderly	
	Left arm	Right arm	Left arm	Right arm
Unimanual				
Short	316	307	412	395*
	129	128	237	245**
Long	322	313	383	373
	186	200	300	309
Bimanual symmetric				
Short	337	334	450	438
	144	147	290	303
Long	347	344	436	423
	204	209	349	358
Bimanual asymmetric				
Short	373	372	486	488
	194	193	344	367
Long	367	365	486	456
	215	217	386	386

Note. Adapted from Stelmach, Amrhein, & Goggin, 1988b, "Age differences in bimanual coordination," *Journal of Gerontology,* **43**, p. 20.
*Top row denotes RT; **Second row denotes MT.

in younger and older adults to study changes in acceleration. They found that the older adults accelerated less rapidly than the young and had a shorter negative acceleration phase. Vrtunski et al. (1984) studied the forces applied in a button press response and found that older adults' release segment contains less braking than young subjects' release segment. They suggest that the well known synchronous relationship between agonist and antagonist muscles is deficient in older adults. Vrtunski and Patterson (1985) found that the forces exerted by older adults in a button press show increased discontinuities in trajectories in comparison to young subjects. This was even more apparent in difficult tasks. In summary, control aspects play a very important role in the production of movements in that older individuals have less control in the production of their movements and fewer control strategies available to them.

CONCLUSION

It is quite apparent that the difficulties experienced by older adults in psychomotor control are partially caused by slowness of response initiation (RT) and response execution (MT). Thus, central mechanisms are responsible for the slowing of RT, and most of the slowing can be linked to a specific deficit. However, these are only a few of the primary mechanisms responsible for the psychomotor decline with advanced age. In order to fully understand the decline, we must examine a continuum of activity which includes physiological, social, health, and behavioral factors. Too often researchers have only concentrated on their specialization and have not acknowledged the involvement of other systems as partially responsible for the deficits in human performance with advanced age. According to Mortimer, Pirozzolo, and Maletta (1982), it is of immediate and future interest to examine the interaction of different hierarchical levels of sensory–motor integration, and to study motor behavior in several different contexts in older individuals. One must consider that a decrease in available strategies is likely to produce deficits in motor performance that may be compensated in different ways depending on task demands.

REFERENCES

BOUISETT, S., & Zattara, M. (1981). A sequence of postural movements precedes voluntary movement. *Neuroscience Letters, 22*, 263-270.

CERELLA, J. (1985). Information processing rates in the elderly. *Psychological Bulletin, 98*, 67-83.

CLARKSON, P.M. (1978). The effect of age and activity level on simple and choice fractionated response time. *European Journal of Applied Physiology, 40*, 17-25.

GOGGIN, N.L., & Christina, R.W. (1979). Reaction time analysis of programmed control of short, rapid aiming movements. *Research Quarterly, 50*, 360-368.

GOGGIN, N.L., & Stelmach, G.E. (1988). *A kinematic analysis of precued movements in young and elderly subjects.* Manuscript in preparation.

GOTTSDANKER, R. (1980a). Aging and the use of advance probability information. *Journal of Motor Behavior, 12*, 133-143.

GOTTSDANKER, R. (1980b). Aging and the maintenance of preparation. *Experimental Aging Research, 6*, 13-27.

GOTTSDANKER, R. (1982). Age and simple reaction time. *Journal of Gerontology, 37*, 342-348.

JORDAN, T.C., & Rabbitt, P.M. (1977). Response times to stimuli of increasing complexity as a function of ageing. *British Journal of Psychology, 68*, 189-201.

LARISH, D.D., & Stelmach, G.E. (1982). Preprogramming, programming, and reprogramming of aimed hand movements as a function of age. *Journal of Motor Behavior, 14*, 322-340.

MANKOVSKII, N.B., Mints, A.Y., & Lysenyuk, V.P. (1980). Regulation of the preparatory period for complex voluntary movement in old and extreme old age. *Human Physiology, 6*, 47-50.

MORTIMER, J.A., Pirozzolo, F.J., & Maletta, G.J. (1982). Overview of the aging motor system. In J. Mortimer, F. Pirozzolo, & G. Maletta (Eds.), *Aging motor system* (pp. 1-6). New York: Praeger.

MURRELL, K.F., & Entwisle, D.G. (1960). Age differences in movement pattern. *Nature, 185*, 948-949.

OCHS, A.L., Newberry, J., Lenhardt, M.L., & Harkins, S.W. (1985). Neural and vestibular aging associated with falls. In J.E. Birren & K.W. Schaie (Eds.), *Handbook of the psychology of aging* (pp. 378-399). New York: Van Nostrand Reinhold.

RABBITT, P.M. (1979). How old and young subjects monitor and control responses for accuracy and speed. *British Journal of Psychology, 70*, 305-311.

RABBITT, P.M. (1982). Breakdown of control processes in old age. In T.M. Field, A. Huston, H.C. Quay, L. Troll, & G. Finley (Eds.), *Review of human development* (pp. 551-568). New York: John Wiley & Sons.

SALTHOUSE, T.A. (1979). Adult age and the speed–accuracy trade-off. *Ergonomics, 22*, 811-821.

SALTHOUSE, T.A. (1985). Speed of behavior and its implications for cognition. In J.E. Birren & K.W. Schaie (Eds.), *Handbook of the psychology of aging* (pp. 400-426). New York: Van Nostrand Reinhold.

SALTHOUSE, T.A., & Somberg, B.L. (1982). Skilled performance: The effects of adult age and experience on elementary processes. *Journal of Experimental Psychology: General, 111*, 176-207.

SPIRDUSO, W.W. (1982). Physical fitness in relation to motor aging. In J. Mortimer, F. Pirozzolo, & G. Maletta (Eds.), *Aging motor system* (pp. 120-151). New York: Praeger.

STELMACH, G.E., Amrhein, P.C., & Goggin, N.L. (1988a). *Maintenance and restructuring of motor preparation with age*. Manuscript in preparation.

STELMACH, G.E., Amrhein, P.C., & Goggin, N.L. (1988b). Age differences in bimanual coordination. *Journal of Gerontology, 43*, 18-23.

STELMACH, G.E., Goggin, N.L., & Amrhein, P.C. (1988). Aging and reprogramming: The restructuring of planned movements. *Psychology and Aging, 3*, 151-157.

STELMACH, G.E., Goggin, N.L., & Garcia-Colera, A. (1987). Movement specification time with age. *Experimental Aging Research, 13*, 39-46.

STELMACH, G.E., & Worringham, C.J. (1985). Sensorimotor deficits related to postural stability. *Clinics in Geriatric Medicine, 1*, 679-694.

SZAFRAN, J. (1951). Changes with age and exclusion of vision in performance at an aiming task. *Quarterly Journal of Experimental Psychology, 3*, 111-118.

VRTUNSKI, P.B., & Patterson, M.B. (1985). Psychomotor decline can be described by discontinuities in response trajectories. *International Journal of Neuroscience, 27*, 265-275.

VRTUNSKI, P.B., Patterson, M.B., & Hill, G.O. (1984). Factor analysis of choice reaction time in young and elderly subjects. *Perceptual and Motor Skills, 59*, 659-676.

WARABI, T., Noda, H., & Kato, T. (1986). Effects of aging on sensorimotor functions of eye and hand movements. *Experimental Neurology, 92*, 686-697.

WEISS, A.D. (1965). The locus of reaction time change with set, motivation, age. *Journal of Gerontology, 20*, 60-64.

WELFORD, A.T. (1969). Speed and accuracy of movement and their changes with age. *Acta Psychologica, 30*, 3-15.

WELFORD, A.T. (1977). Motor performance. In J.E. Birren & K.W. Schaie (Eds.), *Handbook of the psychology of aging* (pp. 450-496). New York: Van Nostrand Reinhold.

WELFORD, A.T. (1981). Signal, noise, performance and age. *Human Factors, 23*, 91-109.

WELFORD, A.T. (1982). Motor skills and aging. In J. Mortimer, F. Pirozzolo, & G. Maletta (Eds.), *Aging motor system* (pp. 152-187). New York: Praeger.

WELFORD, A.T. (1984a). Between bodily changes and performance: Some possible reasons for slowing with age. *Experimental Aging Research, 10*, 73-88.

WELFORD, A.T. (1984b). Psychomotor performance. In C. Eisdorfer (Ed.), *Annual review of gerontology and geriatrics* (pp. 237-273). New York: Springer.

WOOLLACOTT, M.H., Shumway-Cook, A., & Nashner, L. (1982). Postural reflexes and aging. In J. Mortimer, F. Pirozzolo, & G. Maletta (Eds.), *Aging motor system* (pp. 98-119). New York: Praeger.

Acknowledgment

The preparation of this manuscript was supported by a grant from the National Institute on Aging, AG05445.

The Aging Motor System: Skeletal Muscle Weakness

Elsworth R. Buskirk and Steven S. Segal
The Pennsylvania State University

As we age, we tend to modify our lifestyle to the extent that we generally become less physically active. Attempts to counter this trend are only partially successful in all but the most diligent adherents to a regular exercise program. Accordingly, both maximal static and dynamic strength plus maximal speed and power are reduced. These changes have been reviewed by several authors, including Asmussen and Heebold-Nielsen (1961), Shock (1977), Skinner, Tipton, and Vailas (1982), Buskirk (1985), and Green (1986). Nevertheless, there still remains considerable uncertainty with respect to changing strength characteristics with aging in various populations of subjects, the time course of these changes, the separate impact of gender, the effect of physical inactivity, the influence of regular exercise of different types and intensities, and the impact of disability and disease. The focus here is to summarize representative cross-sectional and longitudinal appraisals of strength, endurance, and power in relation to aging, and to relate these changes to the structural and functional changes that occur in aging skeletal muscle.

PERFORMANCE OF COMMON ACTIVITIES

The National Health Interview Survey (NHIS) is conducted in approximately 42,000 households each year by U.S. Bureau of the Census interviewers. In 1984, a special Supplement on Aging (SOA) was designed to collect information about physical limitations as well as other health-related and social information. Although the estimates of the prevalence of disability were based on the simple responses of yes or no, the sample was sufficiently large to provide useful approximations of the prevalence of disability in the U.S. (National Center for Health Statistics, 1987, No. 136).

In general, a greater percentage of women than men had difficulty performing work-associated activities. Two examples are provided in Tables 1 and 2. The sex difference in work performance was largest with lifting or carrying loads, whereas the sex difference was minimal with respect to walking.

Subjective difficulty of performance increased with age, as did the percent of those unable to perform the respective task. People who were employed were less likely than retired people to have difficulty with a task—the proportion

Table 1

Percent of People 55–74 Years of Age Who Have Worked Since Age 45 With Difficulty or Inability to Lift or Carry 25 Pounds

Sample	Age			
	55–59	60–64	65–69	70–74
Men				
Difficulty	11.6	15.4	16.8	23.1
Unable	3.5	3.8	5.6	7.5
Women				
Difficulty	22.9	31.0	33.8	40.8
Unable	9.1	8.7	9.3	10.7

Note. Adapted from NCHS Advanced Data Report Number 136, 1987.

Table 2

Percent of People 55–74 Years of Age Who Have Worked Since Age 45 With Difficulty or Inability to Walk 1/4 Mile

Sample	Age			
	55–59	60–64	65–69	70–74
Men				
Difficulty	12.3	17.0	20.1	23.3
Unable	5.0	7.9	9.4	8.7
Women				
Difficulty	12.6	15.8	19.9	26.6
Unable	5.8	8.0	7.9	10.2

Note. Adapted from NCHS Advanced Data Report Number 136, 1987.

of people experiencing difficulty was two to three times higher among those who had retired. Those who retired for reasons of ill health were the most likely to have difficulty with an activity. Approximately 24% of elderly people have difficulty with heavy housework (Table 3). Obviously, muscular strength and endurance are important for the performance of such activity. At all ages over 65 years, women were significantly more likely than men to have difficulty performing home management activities, but men were also less likely to perform such activities on a regular basis in a household in which women reside (National Center for Health Statistics, 1987, No. 133).

Table 3

**Percent of Persons 65 Years of Age and Over
Who Have Difficulty Doing Heavy Housework**

	Age				
Sample	65–69	70–74	75–79	80–84	85 & over
Men	9.8	13.0	14.6	18.9	33.3
Women	21.8	27.3	33.2	41.7	54.2

Note. Adapted from NCHS Advanced Data Report Number 133, 1987.

The elderly have been described as generally satisfied with their physical fitness, yet they underestimate their ability to exercise (Conrad, 1976). Similarly, McAvoy (1976) found that among those 65 and older, the barrier to regular recreational exercise was their perceived lack of physical ability. Sidney and Shephard (1977) observed that the physical fitness of elderly city dwellers was average or below average, but they perceived themselves as having adequate physical activity. Thus, perception and reality with respect to regular exercise among the elderly are quite different, and the difference may be as great for strength-developing activities as for those involving respiratory–cardiovascular fitness. A key issue would appear to be the improvement of perception of physical ability through education and the modification of fitness, including muscular strength, through a change in lifestyle involving regular exercise.

MUSCLE STRENGTH AND POWER

Assessment of Strength and Power

Strength involves the force developed by contracting muscles, whereas power involves the application of that force per unit of time. Conceptually, power involves both strength and speed. Since strength declines with age as a result of changes within skeletal muscle, power will also decline, but the decline in power is magnified because speed is also compromised due to reductions in nerve conduction velocity and synaptic transmission. These changes may occur in concert with a decrease in the speed of contraction of type II fibers and the increase in the excitability threshold of muscle.

That power does decrease dramatically with aging is illustrated by the results of age-group competition in such events as the shot put, discus throw, vertical jump, and long jump. Training for such competition does not prevent this substantial decline, although it can be rationally argued that the master's athlete seldom devotes the time or achieves the training intensity of the younger athlete.

A variety of measures have been used to document a decrement in the mechanical performance of skeletal muscle with advancing age. Findings reviewed here were obtained from studies of healthy individuals who were not engaged in regular physical exercise. Larsson, Grimby, and Karlsson (1979) evaluated muscle performance of knee extensors using an isokinetic dynamometer (Cybex Div. of Lumex, Inc., Ronkonkoma, NY 11779) in 114 subjects varying in age from 11 to 70 years. These investigators found that the maximum isometric strength, extension velocity, and dynamic strength all increased through the age of 29 years, remained fairly stable through the age of 40, then declined progressively between the ages of 40 and 70 years. In a similarly wide age range of subjects, Bosco and Komi (1980) tested the ability to perform vertical jumps against a force platform (Table 4). Findings indicated that contractile force, power, and the elastic characteristics of leg muscles increase through age 20, and then decrease progressively between 20 and 80 years of age. Similar trends were observed in both male and female subjects, with males being stronger at each age.

Murray, Gardner, Mollinger, and Sepic (1980) measured the static and dynamic contractions (both flexion and extension) in men aged 20 to 86 years and observed a profound decline (Table 5). Murray, Duthic, Gambert, Sepic, and Mollinger (personal communication, 1984) followed the study on men with one on women and found similar strength losses. Knee muscle strength (torque) was assessed during maximum isometric and dynamic (isokinetic) contractions in three groups of healthy women ($N=24$ per group, 20 to 86 years of age). Strength of those in the oldest group ranged from 56 to 78% of that in the youngest group, depending on knee joint position. During isokinetic contractions performed at $36° \cdot s^{-1}$ strength was about 50% greater for knee extension than for flexion. For both actions, torque generated at 30° was usually lower than that generated at 45° or 60°. Maximum strength values were greater for isometric than for isokinetic contractions. Interestingly, knee muscle strength of the women averaged 74% of that of the men, and the decrement in strength from the youngest to the oldest groups was also less for the women than the men (women -22 to -44%; men -35 to -55%). This observation may well be related to the lesser decline in body cell mass with age in women compared to men (Forbes & Reina, 1970).

Table 4

Force and Power Developed During Squatting Jump in Male Age Groups

Age group (yrs)	N	Body weight (kg)	Average force (N)	Average power (W) $W \cdot leg^{-1} kg\ body\ wt^{-1}$
4–6	10	18 ± 2	114 ± 40	16 ± 4
13–17	19	56 ± 9	402 ± 92	22 ± 3
18–28	35	80 ± 10	618 ± 137	23 ± 4
29–40	16	79 ± 7	508 ± 153	17 ± 4
41–49	18	77 ± 12	435 ± 96	14 ± 3
54–65	4	76 ± 12	320 ± 23	19 ± 4
71–73	11	74 ± 8	315 ± 118	7 ± 3

Note. Data are mean ± standard deviation. Adapted from Bosco & Komi, 1980.

Table 5

Isometric Knee Flexor and Extensor Muscle Strength (kg-cm)

Age group (yrs)	N	Flexor strength in 3 knee joint positions			Extensor strength in 3 knee joint positions		
		30[o,b,c]	45[o,b,c]	60[o,a,b,c]	30[o,b]	45[o,a,b,c]	60[o,a,b,c]
20–35	24	719 ± 37	792 ± 38	792 ± 36	1188 ± 58	1724 ± 83	1797 ± 69
42-61	24	682 ± 38	721 ± 40	676 ± 39	1056 ± 60	1444 ± 69	1402 ± 65
70-86	24	502 ± 33	510 ± 32	505 ± 31	903 ± 45	1110 ± 68	1124 ± 56

Note. Data are mean ± SEM. Adapted from Murray et al., 1984.
[a]Youngest different from middle-aged ($p < .01$). [b]Youngest different from oldest ($p < .01$).
[c]Middle-aged different from oldest ($p < .01$).

The findings of greater isometric strength than isokinetic strength for knee extension has been observed by others in addition to Murray and her colleagues (e.g., Osternig, 1975; Smidt, 1973; Thorstensson, Grimby, & Karlsson, 1976). An inherent feature of muscle is that force development is lower as velocity of contraction increases (Close, 1972), perhaps because less time is available for the formation of cross-bridges as the muscle fibers shorten—a property that may be further modified by aging or disuse.

In a comparison between two age groups, Davies, White, and Young (1983) measured the ability of older (60 ± 1 yr) and younger (22 ± 1 yr) men to develop power during performance both with the vertical jump and during cycling, and found substantial decrements in contractile force and power output in the leg muscles of older subjects. Indirect (surface electrodes) electrical stimulation of the triceps surae muscle indicated that maximal force production of the plantar flexors was 50–60% of that obtained for younger men, and that the muscles of older men both contracted and relaxed more slowly (Davies & White, 1983; Davies et al., 1983). The fact that strength differences between age groups persisted during electrical stimulation supports the idea of changes in skeletal muscle tissue, as opposed to a change in the ability to recruit muscle fibers.

Body Composition, Age, and Strength

The relationship between size and strength of the quadriceps muscle group was determined in older (71–81 yrs) and younger (20–29 yrs) women (Young, Stokes, & Crowe, 1984). Force production was measured using knee extension, and muscle cross-sectional area was determined by planimetry of photographs taken of transverse ultrasound scans of the thigh. It was found that the decline in quadriceps strength in the older subjects could be explained by a proportional decline in the size of this muscle group. The results from this study suggested that there was no difference in the intrinsic contractile strength of aged muscle, a concept that has received general support (Grimby & Saltin, 1983; Saltin & Gollnick, 1983).

In apparent conflict with the concept of constant force production per muscle cross-sectional area was the finding by Larsson et al. (1979) that a significant reduction in knee extensor strength was not accompanied by a reduction in thigh girth. These authors postulated that in aged subjects, muscle tissue may be replaced with fat and connective tissue. It is interesting to note that, using a rat model, Segal, Faulkner, and White (1986) found a reduction in specific tension (force per muscle cross-sectional area) of the soleus muscle following transplantation, a change that was in fact accounted for by the increase in extracellular fluid volume and connective tissue protein content. These observations collectively support the concept that the force per cross-sectional area of *functional contractile protein* remains virtually constant. With aging, any loss in contractile protein in conjunction with an increase in noncontractile tissue elements would decrease the force production per cross-sectional area of a limb, and thereby decrease apparent muscle strength. With loss of muscle tissue alone, a proportional reduction in force production and both muscle and limb cross-sectional area would be observed.

Several investigators have shown that total body potassium content (^{40}K assessment) declines with age (Borkan, Hults, Gerzof, Robbins, & Silbert, 1983; Bruce, Andersson, Arvidsson, & Isaksson, 1980; Cohn et al., 1980), which has been taken as an indication of the loss of body cell mass. Cohn et al. (1980), using neutron-activation analysis for total body nitrogen, suggested that the loss of muscle mass in the elderly is greater than the loss of nonmuscle lean tissue. Borkan et al. (1983), using computed tomography, found less lean tissue in the upper arm, abdomen, and thigh in older subjects, together with greater fat content within and between muscles. Other investigators have found from muscle biopsies that intramuscular fat, connective tissue, and lipofuscin granules accumulate in subjects 60 to 96 years of age along with fiber atrophy, particularly in type II fibers (Scelsi, Marchetti, & Poggi, 1980; Shafiq, Lewis, Dimino, & Schutta, 1978; Tomonaga, 1977).

As shown by several other body composition studies, body cell mass decreases among the elderly. Steen (1988) recently reviewed these studies and cites the observation that by age 70, human skeletal muscle has lost 40% of its maximal weight in early adult life, whereas other tissues lose 20% or less. Steen cites his and his colleagues' work in which by the eighth decade of life body cell mass has decreased about two kg in men, but much less in women. Total body water tended to decrease in the two sexes in a pattern similar to that of body cell mass.

Anatomical Location

The magnitude of the effects of aging on skeletal muscle function may vary with the muscle group and anatomical location. In a comparison of the effects of aging on the mechanical properties of arm and leg muscles, McDonagh, White, and Davies (1984) tested two groups of men, 71 (±4) and 26 (±6) years old, respectively. They found that maximum voluntary contraction of the older men was 41% lower in the triceps surae and 20% lower in the elbow flexors, compared to values obtained from the younger men. Similar differences in contractile strength with anatomical location were found using indirect electrical stimulation of muscles, again indicating that the changes observed with aging were specific to the muscle tissue rather than to differences in the subjects' ability to recruit muscle fibers.

Studies using electrical stimulation of muscle (McDonagh et al., 1984) also revealed that the slowing of contraction and relaxation times observed in the triceps surae did not occur in the elbow flexors. To explain the greater loss of strength and the relative slowing of the leg muscles, these authors proposed that, with age, leg muscle activity is primarily postural and associated with slow walking. Standing and slow walking will preferentially recruit slow, or type I, muscle fibers and will not require recruitment of the larger and faster contracting type II muscle fibers (Burke, 1981). In contrast, the arms continue to perform rapid movements, which will involve type II muscle fiber contraction (Burke, 1981) and tend to preserve this fiber type.

Eddinger, Cassens, and Moss (1986) used fiber bundles and skinned single fiber preparations to determine the contractile properties of characteristically slow-twitch (soleus) and fast-twitch (extensor digitorum longus, EDL) muscles in young (9 months) and old (30 months) rats. Maximum shortening velocity was unchanged in the EDL muscle but increased in the soleus muscle. Maximal force production increased in soleus muscle fibers, yet was unchanged in EDL muscle preparations. Calcium sensitivity of the contractile apparatus was unaffected by age in both fiber types. These data raise the question of whether there may be intrinsic fiber-type specific differences in the muscular adaptations that occur with aging.

Strength Development and Preservation

It has been commonly reported that regular resistance exercise produces increased strength in the elderly (Chapman, deVries, & Swezey, 1972; Daykin, 1967; Moritani & deVries, 1981; Rodriques, DePalma, & Daykin, 1965). Hettinger (1961) reviewed several studies on males and females 6 to 65 years of age with respect to their strength development with regular exercise. He concluded that by the sixth decade men and women were roughly equal in ability and could gain strength at the rate of 30 to 40% of that demonstrated by 20- to 30-year-old men. Barry, Steinmet, Page, and Rodahl (1966) reported that older men and women who engaged in a 3-month calisthenic and cycle ergometer program demonstrated significant increases in power as measured by a vertical jump.

Moritani and deVries (1981) suggested that older men gain strength largely through recruitment of more motor units, whereas younger men gain strength through muscle hypertrophy. Larsson (1982) and Aniansson and Gustafsson (1981) suggest that older men can achieve muscle hypertrophy with regular resistance exercise.

There are numerous examples of the preservation of strength in later life. A recent one is that described by Dummer, Vaccaro, and Clarke (1985), who evaluated the strength and flexibility of two women who competed in master's swimming events. Their respective ages were 70 and 71 years. Although the authors cite a general lack of comparative data, they concluded that the women had greater strength than less active women of comparable age and scored well within the range for physically fit women who were considerably younger. Measurements made included grip strength plus shoulder and knee flexion and extension. More important, both women felt free to complete all strength tests at maximal levels and through a full range of motion—they had confidence in their abilities in this regard.

To summarize, it appears that strength peaks in the third decade, followed by a fairly level trend through age 40 or 50, about a 20% loss to the mid-60s, with a subsequent further decline in later years (Larsson, 1982; Montoye & Lamphiear, 1977). Both dynamic and isometric strength are affected in men and women (Young et al., 1984, 1985). There is evidence that leg strength declines more rapidly than grip or arm strength (Grimby & Saltin, 1983; McDonagh et al., 1984; Simonson, 1947), but strength changes may well be occupationally and recreationally dependent, that is, those who use their strength on a regular basis preserve it more effectively (Petrofsky & Lind, 1975). Maximum power generated in the 30s has been found to decrease about 6% per decade during ergometer cycling (Makrides, Heigenhauser, McCartney, & Jones, 1985). A strong argument can be made that interindividual differences are relatively large with respect to the rate and extent of the functional decline in strength with aging, although such decline is eventually inevitable.

MUSCULAR ENDURANCE

A priori, it can be stated that if the maximal strength and mass of a muscle is decreased with age, then the muscle will fatigue more readily. This is because a given absolute load will represent a greater relative percentage of maximal load in the smaller muscle, which will therefore have to work at a higher percentage of its capacity compared to a larger muscle (Close, 1972). During physical exercise, a given absolute work rate will require a greater percentage of maximal aerobic power in older persons, which will contribute to a greater rate of fatigue (Grimby & Saltin, 1983).

The energy metabolism of skeletal muscle apparently becomes less effective at sustaining contractile function with aging. Electrical stimulation of the triceps surae in humans, using intermittent tetanic trains for a 2-minute period, resulted in a greater relative loss of tension in older subjects, indicating their greater susceptibility to fatigue (Davies & White, 1983). Using rats, Dudley and Fleck (1984) performed in situ stimulation of soleus and gastrocnemius muscles in young (7 month) and old (23 month) rats, and measured the tissue concentrations of selected metabolites at rest and at the end of a fatigue protocol. Fatigued muscle samples from aged rats were found to have lower concentrations of phosphocreatine and ATP, as well as higher concentrations of lactate. Since young and old muscles had similar metabolite concentrations at rest, these changes were interpreted to reflect a reduced ability of aged muscle to maintain energy balance during muscular exercise, particularly in the ability to regenerate ATP.

Two primary factors influence the ability of skeletal muscle to perform aerobically for sustained periods of time: the delivery of oxygen by the cardiovascular system, and oxygen consumption by mitochondria in the tissue. Each factor has been investigated with respect to the greater fatigability of aged muscle. Using in situ stimulation of the plantar flexors, it was observed that muscles from senescent (24 month) rats underwent a greater fatigue than those of younger (12 month) animals, and that this was associated with lower muscle blood flows during contractions (Irion, Vasthare, & Tuma, 1987). Additionally, lower maximal blood flows were obtained in aged rats during pharmacologically induced vasodilation, indicating that the potential to increase muscle blood flow during exercise was significantly lower in older animals.

The reduced tissue perfusion in aged muscles can explain the higher lactate and lower high-energy phosphate concentrations (Dudley & Fleck, 1984), being ascribable to greater reliance on glycolysis and impaired oxidative phosporylation in the presence of diminished oxygen delivery. The lower blood flow would also decrease the washout of metabolic products (lactate, carbon dioxide), which may in turn directly contribute to fatigue by affecting intramuscular pH and contractile protein function. These effects of blood flow on skeletal muscle function serve to illustrate that muscular endurance is intimately associated with cardiovascular function.

Mitochondria are the site of oxygen consumption in muscle cells (Saltin & Gollnick, 1983). Farrar, Martin, and Ardies (1981) isolated mitochondria from the gastrocnemious-plantaris muscle group of rats up to 720 days old. With aging of the rats, these investigators found a loss of mitochondrial protein in muscle fibers, with no change in the mitochondrial respiratory characteristics. Run conditioning (1 hr • d^{-1}, 25 m • min^{-1}) attenuated the loss of mitochondrial protein with aging, yet did not prevent aging muscle from undergoing significant atrophy (Farrar et al., 1981). Orlander, Kiessling, Larsson, Karlsson, and Aniansson (1978) studied biopsy samples of human vastus lateralis muscles in a group of 69 subjects ranging in age from 16 to 76 years and found that aging was associated with a significant reduction in the fraction of muscle cellular volume occupied by mitochondria, yet it did not affect the specific activity of mitochondrial enzymes. These morphological and biochemical data from human tissues support the loss of mitochondrial protein (Farrer et al., 1981) and reduction in cytochrome-c concentration (Dudley & Fleck, 1984) with aging in rats.

The reduction in tissue oxidative capacity (Farrer et al., 1981) and reduced oxygen delivery (Irion et al., 1987), coupled with the loss of contractile protein discussed above, collectively support the proposal that aging muscle has an impaired ability for prolonged muscular activity (Ermini, 1976). In contrast to declines in strength, however, muscular endurance during low and moderate contraction intensities declines little with age until senescence begins to play a role (Aniansson, Grimby, Hedberg, Rungren, & Sperling, 1978; Larsson et al., 1979).

MUSCLE FIBERS: SIZE, NUMBER, TYPE, AND ULTRASTRUCTURE

Muscular atrophy accompanying aging can be attributable to a loss of muscle fibers, atrophy of existing fibers, or both (Green, 1986). A change in the fiber composition of skeletal muscles can occur either by selective loss of a particular fiber type or by conversion of one fiber type to another, as would occur during the process of denervation and reinnervation (Buller, Eccles, & Eccles, 1960; Carlson, 1981).

Many studies of aging human muscle have used needle biopsy to obtain tissue for analysis. Orlander et al. (1978) biopsied the vastus lateralis in men aged 16 to 76 years. Using myofibrillar ATPase activity to differentiate between type I (acid stable) and type II (alkaline stable) fibers (slow- and fast-twitch fibers, respectively), they observed a significant increase in the proportion of type I fibers with age. Using similar techniques, Larsson (1978) and Larsson et al. (1979) also found a reduction in the proportion of type II fibers of vastus lateralis muscles with aging (Table 6) that was correlated with the loss of muscle strength measured in the same subjects from which biopsies were obtained. Subsequent biopsy studies confirmed an altered fiber type distribution and decreased fiber area

Table 6

Vastus Lateralis m. Fiber Areas and Fiber Area Ratios of Different Age Groups: Needle Biopsy, Lesser Fiber Diameter Method

		Area		Area ratio
Group (yrs)	N	Type I	Type II	Type II/I
		(μm^2 $\cdot$ 10^2)		
20-29	11	29.5 $\pm$ 2.5	36.6 $\pm$ 2.2	1.28 $\pm$ 0.07
30-39	12	29.2 $\pm$ 1.5	36.7 $\pm$ 2.9	1.27 $\pm$ 0.09
40-49	10	31.9 $\pm$ 1.9	32.6 $\pm$ 2.4	1.03 $\pm$ 0.06
50-59	12	28.8 $\pm$ 1.6	28.0 $\pm$ 1.2	0.99 $\pm$ 0.05
60-65	10	22.6 $\pm$ 2.4	21.2 $\pm$ 1.7	0.99 $\pm$ 0.09

Note. Data are mean $\pm$ SEM. Adapted from Larsson, 1978.

occurring between the third and seventh decade, characterized by a decline in the relative occurrence and preferential atrophy of type II fibers (Larsson, 1983).

In a comparison of biopsies of vastus lateralis and biceps brachii in men and women 78–81 years old, muscle fiber atrophy was found to be more common in women, perhaps attributable to less habitual physical activity relative to men (Grimby, Danneskiold-Samsoe, Hvid, & Saltin, 1982). Changes in fiber type were greater in the vastus lateralis than in the biceps brachii muscles, there being a greater loss of type II fibers in the vastus. These investigators also used measurements of body cell mass, coupled with anthropomorphic data, to suggest that much of the loss in muscle mass is due to the loss of muscle fibers.

Other investigators have reported that the relative occurrence of fiber types does not change with age (cf. Green, 1986). There are several possible reasons for this discrepancy. Lexell, Taylor, and Sjöstrom (1985) have shown that a single needle biopsy is a poor estimator of the fiber type proportion for the whole muscle. Instead, several biopsies from different regions of a muscle should be analyzed to obtain more accurate representation (Lexell et al., 1985). Also, the size and location of biopsy samples may differ between studies. Larger tissue samples containing a greater number of muscle fibers (obtained by using open biopsy procedures), are more representative of the fiber type distribution in a muscle when compared to the more typical (and less traumatic) percutaneous needle biopsies. Biopsy material taken at a similar depth for all subjects may actually represent deeper regions of an older, atrophied muscle. Differences in physical activity between age groups can also lead to erroneous conclusions in cross-sectional studies of the effects of aging on muscle fiber type. For example, younger more active subjects would tend to have greater proportions of the oxidative type I and type IIA fiber types (Saltin & Gollnick, 1983) compared to older, relatively inactive subjects.

Lexell, Henriksson-Larsén, Winblad, and Sjöstrom (1983) obtained intact muscles from human cadavers that had no history of neuromuscular disease. By adapting conventional preparative procedures to accommodate larger tissue samples, Lexell (1983) obtained data that were representative of entire muscle cross sections (Table 7). The calculated total number of type I and type II muscle fibers (as identified by the myofibrillar ATPase reaction) of entire vastus lateralis muscle cross sections were compared from men of two age groups: 71 (± 1) years and 30 (± 6) years. The findings indicated that muscle size and fiber number were reduced proportionally (by 18 and 25%, respectively) in older muscles, with no change in the size of individual muscle fibers. There was no significant change in the proportion of fiber types. These results suggested that the reduction in muscle volume with increasing age is due to the reduction in the total number of fibers, with no reduction in fiber size.

In direct contrast to these findings in human muscle are the results of Eddinger, Moss, and Cassens (1985), who counted the total number of fibers in soleus and extensor digitorum longus muscle cross sections of rats aged 3 to 30 months and observed no loss of muscle fibers with aging. Nor was a change found in fiber type distribution, an observation that was consistent with the results of Lexell et al. (1983) obtained from human muscle. Thus, the mode of muscle atrophy with aging may differ between species, with greater loss of muscle fibers occurring in humans than in rats.

Two different phenomena may account for the loss of muscle fibers with age. Muscle fibers may become injured and eliminated, or may degenerate in response to denervation. Satellite cells are intimately involved in the growth of normal muscle and the repair of damaged muscle (Carlson & Faulkner, 1983). In injured muscle, surviving satellite cells are activated to become the myogenic stem cells that recapitulate ontogenic events in order to repair or replace damaged muscle fibers (Carlson & Faulkner, 1983). Schultz and Lipton (1982) determined the proliferative potential of satellite cells in relation to the age of the host organism. Satellite cells were obtained from leg muscles of rats ranging from 6 days to 30 months of age, and the cells were grown in culture. Under identical in vitro conditions, the ability of satellite cells to proliferate was inversely proportional to the age of the donor animal (Schultz & Lipton, 1982). Thus, the limited prolifer-

Table 7

Vastus Lateralis m. Fiber Size, Number, and Type of Two Age Groups: Whole Muscle Cross-Section Method

Group (yrs)	N	No. of fibers per mm²	Total no. of fibers	Proportion of type I fibers
30 ± 6	6	146 ± 14	478,000 ± 56,000	51 ± 3
72 ± 1	6	136 ± 20	364,000 ± 50,000	54 ± 5
Young vs. old		n.s.	$p < 0.01$	n.s.

Note. Data are mean ± standard deviation. Adapted from Lexell, Henriksson-Larsén, Winblad, and Sjöstrom, 1983.

ative capacity of satellite cells in aged animals may contribute to atrophic changes in skeletal muscle accompanying aging.

Tomonaga (1977) studied muscle biopsies obtained from 79 patients 60–90 years old who had no neuromuscular disease. With light microscopy, a generalized atrophy of fibers was observed, particularly of type II fibers, as was the presence of centralized nuclei. With electron microscopy, the sarcomere appeared to be disorganized, with streaming of Z-bands, and abnormal muscle nuclei and satellite cells were observed. Note that these changes in muscle ultrastructure are classic signs of muscle fiber degeneration and regeneration (Carlson & Faulkner, 1983). Tomonaga (1977) attributed most of these changes to neuropathic processes (cf. Carlson, 1981) and suggested that various factors act at many levels, including the motor neuron, peripheral nerves, motor endplates, and the muscle cell, to induce the neuropathic and myopathic changes seen in the muscles of the aged.

It appears that if denervation of muscle fibers occurs, and these fibers are subsequently reinnervated, muscle mass and strength are preserved. Brown (1973) used electrophysiological techniques to estimate the number and size of the thenar muscle motor units in 61 control subjects ranging in age from 9 to 89 years and having no history of neuromuscular disease. There was a slight decrease in the number of motor units between the ages of 9 and 60. After age 60, however, there was a sharp drop in motor unit number. Beyond the sixth decade, many subjects had fewer than half of the number of motor units they'd had in youth. Despite the loss of motor units, the strength and size of the thenar musculature was maintained, attributable to a significant increase in motor unit size (Brown, 1973). This functional compensation may be attributable to reinnervation of denervated muscle fibers by sprouting from adjacent, healthy motor axons. During aging, the increase in larger motor units, coupled with the loss of smaller motor units, would be predicted to result in a diminution of fine motor control (Burke, 1981). This hypothesis has yet to be tested directly.

Needle biopsies of vastus lateralis and biceps brachii in men and women 78–81 years old revealed the presence of "enclosed" fibers (muscle fibers surrounded by others of similar type) in most of the samples obtained (Grimby et al., 1982). Such fiber type grouping (adjacent fibers of similar metabolic and contractile properties) virtually never occurs in young healthy humans; rather, the territory of fibers comprising a motor unit is dispersed (Burke, 1981). The extent to which fiber type grouping occurs in aging muscle varies with muscle location, being more common in the vastus lateralis than in the biceps brachii (Grimby & Saltin, 1983).

This grouping of muscle fibers may be explained by initial denervation of existing fibers (attributable to the loss of corresponding motoneurons in the spinal cord) followed by reinnervation of these fibers via sprouting of axons from adjacent, viable motor nerve fibers (Carlson & Faulkner, 1983; Green, 1986). The change in fiber type that accompanies reinnervation by a "foreign" nerve was first demonstrated in the classic experiments of Buller et al. (1960) and has been subsequently reproduced in many laboratories. If the relative composition of fiber types does not change with loss of motor neurons/motor units during aging, it is likely that the reinnervation of fibers occurs in accord with the existing distribution of type I and type II motoneurons, implying that each has similar capacity for reinnervation (Grimby & Saltin, 1983).

In summary it appears that, in humans, the reduction in muscle mass with aging may be primarily attributable to a loss of muscle fibers, which in turn may be attributable to both the loss of motoneurons and direct injury to muscle fibers. The factors that determine whether a denervated fiber is either subsequently lost or becomes reinnervated by a viable nerve sprout (and is thereby preserved) are presently undefined. The loss of injured muscle fibers with aging appears to be explained by degeneration coupled with a depressed regenerative capacity. Atrophy of existing muscle fibers can be explained by inactivity and the corresponding lack of fiber recruitment. Both type I and type II fibers appear to be equally susceptible to the aging process; the widespread concept that there is selective loss and atrophy of type II muscle fibers may be attributable to the inherent limitations in the use of needle biopsy and cross-sectional studies to obtain the existing data.

CONCLUSIONS

There is little disagreement that advanced age has deleterious effects on skeletal muscle and physical performance. Changes in skeletal muscle with age include *decreases* in the following:

- Muscle fiber size;
- Muscle fiber number;
- Myofibrillar ATPase activity;
- ATP, creatine phosphate;
- Glycogen, glycolytic enzymes;
- Oxidative enzymes;
- Mitochondrial protein;
- Impulse conduction veocity.

Changes in skeletal muscle with age include *increases* in the following:

- Collagen cross-linking;
- Ratio of Type I/II fibers (?);
- Membrane excitability threshold;
- Connective tissue.

Muscle strength and power increase during normal growth and maturation, plateau and begin to decline during middle age, and diminish progressively with advancing age and senescence. Specific changes in the structure and metabolic properties of muscle can account for much of the decrement in physical performance with aging. Regular exercise can attenuate the magnitude of functional decrements ascribable to the preservation of the contractile and metabolic machinery in skeletal muscle fibers.

Preservation of muscular endurance appears to be favored over preservation of muscle mass and strength. The loss of muscle mass is ascribable to both a decrease in fiber number and atrophy of existing fibers. The atrophy of remaining fibers may be attenuated by regular exercise; however, the muscle fiber loss appears to be due to both a loss of motor neurons centrally and a diminished regenerative capacity of muscle tissue. These latter phenomena appear to be unaffected by exercise, and thus may be considered an inevitable consequence of the aging process.

Attention here has focused on aging in healthy, moderately active men and women. Factors such as nutrition, disability, disease, and mental attitude can certainly modify the time course and magnitude of the aging process and need to be considered in future studies. Most of the existing data have come from cross-sectional comparisons between different subgroups; longitudinal appraisals are sorely needed. We are all faced with the inevitable consequences of aging, yet each of us has the capacity to modify the aging process in our own bodies through appropriate activity and diet.

REFERENCES

ANIANSSON, A., Grimby, G., Hedberg, M., Rungren, A., & Sperling, L. (1978). Muscle function in old age. *Scandinavian Journal of Rehabilitation Medicine, 6*, 43-49.

ANIANSSON, A., & Gustafsson, E. (1981). Physical training in elderly men with special reference to quadriceps muscle strength and morphology. *Clinical Physiology, 1*, 87-98.

ASMUSSEN, E., & Heebold-Nielsen, B. (1961). Isometric muscle strength of adult men and women. In E. Asmussen, A. Fredsted, & E. Ryge (Eds.), *Communications from the testing and observations institute of the Danish national association for infantile paralysis, No. 11*, Copenhagen.

BARRY, A.J., Steinmetz, J.R., Page, H.F., & Rodahl, K. (1966). The effects of physical conditioning on older individuals. II. Motor performance and cognitive function. *Journal of Gerontology, 21*, 192-199.

BORKAN, G.A., Hults, D.E., Gerzof, A.F., Robbins, A.H., & Silbert, C.K. (1983). Age changes in body composition revealed by computer tomography. *Journal of Gerontology, 38*, 363-677.

BOSCO, C., & Komi, P.V. (1980). Influence of aging on the mechanical behavior of leg extensor muscles. *European Journal of Applied Physiology, 43*, 209-219.

BROWN, W.F. (1973). Functional compensation of human motor units in health and disease. *Journal of the Neurological Sciences, 20*, 199-209.

BRUCE, A., Andersson, M., Arvidsson, B., & Isaksson, B. (1980). Body composition. Prediction of normal body potassium, body water and body fat in adults on the basis of body height, body weight and age. *Scandinavian Journal of Clinical Laboratory Investigations, 40*, 461-473.

BULLER, A.J., Eccles, J.C., & Eccles, R.M. (1960). Interactions between motoneurons and muscles in respect of the characteristic speeds of their responses. *Journal of Physiology, 150*, 417-439.

BURKE, R.E. (1981). Motor units: Anatomy, physiology, and functional organization. In V.B. Brooks (Ed.), *Handbook of physiology: The nervous system, Vol. II, motor control* (pp. 345-422). Bethesda, MD: American Physiological Society.

BUSKIRK, E.R. (1985). Health maintenance and longevity: Exercise. In C.E. Finch & E.L. Schneider (Eds.), *Handbook of the biology of aging* (2nd ed.) (pp. 894-931). New York: Van Nostrand Reinhold.

CARLSON, B.M. (1981). Denervation, reinnervation, and regeneration of skeletal muscle. *Otolaryngology Head Neck Surgery,* **89**, 192-196.

CARLSON, B.M., & Faulkner, J.A. (1983). The regeneration of skeletal muscle fibers following injury: A review. *Medicine and Science in Sports and Exercise,* **15**, 187-198.

CHAPMAN, E.A., deVries, H.A., & Swezey, R. (1972). Joint stiffness: Effects of exercise on young and old men. *Journal of Gerontology,* **27**, 218-221.

CLOSE, R.I. (1972). Dynamic properties of mammalian skeletal muscles. *Physiological Reviews,* **52**, 129-197.

COHN, S.H., Vartsky, D., Yasumura, S., Sawitsky, A., Zanzi, I., Vaswani, A., & Ellis, K.J. (1980). Compartmental body composition based on total-body nitrogen, potassium, and calcium. *American Journal of Physiology,* **239**, E524-E530.

CONRAD, C.C. (1976, April 11). When you're young at heart. *Aging.* Washington, DC: Administration on Aging, Department of Health, Education and Welfare.

DAVIES, C.T.M., & White, M.J. (1983). Contractile properties of elderly human triceps surae. *Gerontology,* **29**, 19-25.

DAVIES, C.T.M., White, M.J., & Young, K. (1983). Electrically evoked and voluntary maximal isometric tension in relation to dynamic muscle performance in elderly male subjects, aged 69 years. *European Journal of Applied Physiology,* **51**, 37-43.

DAYKIN, H.P. (1967). The application of isometrics in geriatric treatment. *American Corrective Therapy Journal,* **21**, 203-205.

DUDLEY, G.A., & Fleck, S.J. (1984). Metabolite changes in aged muscle during stimulation. *Journal of Gerontology,* **39**, 183-186.

DUMMER, G.M., Vaccaro, P., & Clarke, D.H. (1985). Muscular strength and flexibility of two female masters swimmers in the eighth decade of life. *Journal of Orthopedics Sports Physical Therapy,* **6**, 235-237.

EDDINGER, T.J., Cassens, R.G., & Moss, R.L. (1986). Mechanical and histochemical characterization of skeletal muscles from senescent rats. *American Journal of Physiology,* **20**, C421-C430.

EDDINGER, T.J., Moss, R.L., & Cassens, R.G. (1985). Fiber number and type compositon in extensor digitorum longus, soleus, and diaphragm muscles with aging in Fisher 344 rats. *The Journal of Histochemistry and Cytochemistry,* **33**, 1033-1041.

ERMINI, M. (1976). Ageing changes in mammalian skeletal muscle. *Gerontology,* **22**, 301-316.

FARRAR, R.P., Martin, T.P., & Ardies, C.M. (1981). The interaction of aging and endurance exercise upon the mitochondrial function of skeletal muscle. *Journal of Gerontology,* **36**, 642-647.

FORBES, G.B., & Reina, J.C. (1970). Adult lean body mass declines with age: Some longitudinal observations. *Metabolism,* **19**, 653-663.

GREEN, H.J. (1986). Characteristics of aging human skeletal muscles. In J.R. Sutton & R.M. Brock (Eds.), *Sports medicine for the mature athlete* (pp. 17-26). Indianapolis: Benchmark Press.

GRIMBY, G., Danneskiold-Samsoe, B., Hvid, K., & Saltin, B. (1982). Morphology and enzymatic capacity in arm and leg muscles in 78-81 year old men and women. *Acta Physiologica Scandinavica,* **115,** 125-134.

GRIMBY, G., & Saltin, B. (1983). The ageing muscle. *Clinical Physiology,* **3,** 209-218.

HETTINGER, T. (1961). *Physiology of strength.* Springfield, IL: Charles C. Thomas.

IRION, G.L., Vasthare, U.S., & Tuma, R.F. (1987). Age-related change in skeletal muscle blood flow in the rat. *Journal of Gerontology,* **42,** 660-665.

LARSSON, L. (1978). Morphological and functional characteristics of the ageing skeletal muscle in man. *Acta Physiologica Scandinavica,* **457** (Suppl.), 1-36.

LARSSON, L. (1982). Physical training effects on muscle morphology in sedentary males at different areas. *Medicine & Science in Sports & Exercise,* **14,** 203-206.

LARSSON, L. (1983). Histochemical characteristics of human skeletal muscle during aging. *Acta Physiological Scandinavica,* **117,** 469-471.

LARSSON, L., Grimby, G., & Karlsson, J. (1979). Muscle strength and speed of movement in relation to age and muscle morphology. *Journal of Applied Physiology: Respiratory Environmental Exercise Physiology,* **46,** 451-456.

LEXELL, J., Henriksson-Larsén, K., Winblad, B., & Sjöstrom, M. (1983). Distribution of different fiber types in human skeletal muscles: Effects of aging studied in whole muscle cross sections. *Muscle & Nerve,* **6,** 588-595.

LEXELL, J., Taylor, C., & Sjöstrom, M. (1985). Analysis of sampling errors in biopsy techniques using data from whole muscle cross sections. *Journal of Applied Physiology,* **59,** 1228-1235.

MAKRIDES, L., Heigenhauser, G.J., McCartney, N., & Jones, N.L. (1985). Maximal short term exercise capacity in healthy subjects aged 15-70 years. *Clinical Science,* **69,** 197-205.

McAVOY, L.H. (1976). *Recreation references of the elderly persons in Minnesota.* Unpublished doctoral dissertation, University of Minnesota.

McDONAGH, M.J.N., White, M.J., & Davies, C.T.M. (1984). Different effects of ageing on the mechanical properties of human arm and leg muscles. *Gerontology,* **30,** 49-54.

MONTOYE, H.J., & Lamphiear, D.E. (1977). Grip and arm strength in males and females, age 10 to 69. *Research Quarterly,* **48,** 109-120.

MORITANI, T., & de Vries, H.A. (1981). Neural factors versus hypertrophy in the time course of muscle strength gain in young and old men. *Journal of Gerontology,* **36,** 294-297.

MURRAY, M.P., Gardner, G.M., Mollinger, L.A., & Sepic, S.B. (1980). Strength of isometric and isokinetic contractions. Knee muscles of men aged 20 to 86. *Physical Therapy,* **60,** 412-419.

NATIONAL Center for Health Statistics. (1987, June 10). Aging in the eighties. Functional limitations of individuals age 65 years and over. *Advance data from vital and health statistics, No. 133.* (DHHS Pub. No. PHS 87-1250). Hyattesville, MD: Public Health Service.

NATIONAL Center for Health Statistics. (1987, May 8). Aging in the eighties. Ability to perform work-related activities. Data from the supplement on aging to the national health interview survey, United States, 1984. *Advance data from vital and health statistics, No. 136.* (DHHS Pub. No. PHS 87-1250). Hyattesville, MD: Public Health Service.

ORLANDER, J., Kiessling, K.-H., Larsson, L., Karlsson, J., & Aniansson, A. (1978). Skeletal muscle metabolism and ultrastructure in relation to age in sedentary men. *Acta Physiological Scandinavica,* **104**, 249-261.

OSTERNIG, L.R. (1975). Optimal isokinetic loads and velocities producing muscular power in human subjects. *Archives of Physical Medicine and Rehabilitation,* **56**, 152-155.

PETROFSKY, J.S., & Lind, A.R. (1975). Aging, isometric strength and endurance and cardiovascular responses to static effort. *Journal of Applied Physiology,* **38**, 91-95.

RODRIQUEZ, M.J., DePalma, J.J., & Daykin, H.P. (1965). Isometric exercise in general practice. *Journal of the Association of Physical and Mental Rehabilitation,* **19**, 197-200.

SALTIN, B., & Gollnick, P.D. (1983). Skeletal muscle adaptability: Significance for metabolism and performance. In V.B. Brooks (Ed.), *Handbook of physiology, section 10: Skeletal muscle* (pp. 555-631). Bethesda, MD: American Physiological Society.

SCELSI, R., Marchetti, C., & Poggi, P. (1980). Histochemical and ultrastructural aspects of M. vastus lateralis in sedentary old people (age 65–89 years). *Acta Neuropathologica,* **51**, 99-105.

SCHULTZ, E., & Lipton, B.H. (1982). Skeletal muscle satellite cells: Changes in proliferation potential as a function of age. *Mechanism of Ageing and Development,* **20**, 377-383.

SEGAL, S.S., Faulkner, J.A., & White, T.P. (1986). Architecture, composition, and contractile properties of rat soleus muscle grafts. *American Journal of Physiology,* **250**, C474-C479.

SHAFIQ, S.A., Lewis, S.G., Dimino, L.C., & Schutta, H.S. (1978). Electron microscopic study of skeletal muscle in eldery subjects. In G. Kaldor & W.J.D. Battista (Eds.), *Aging, vol. 6.* New York: Raven Press.

SHOCK, N.W. (1977). Systems integration. In C. Finch & L. Hayflick (Eds.), *Handbook of the biology of aging* (pp. 639-665). New York: Van Nostrand Reinhold.

SIDNEY, K.H., & Shephard, R.J. (1977). Activity patterns of elderly men and women. *Journal of Gerontology,* **32**, 25-32.

SIMONSON, E. (1947). Physical fitness and work capacity of older men. *Geriatrics,* **2**, 110-119.

SKINNER, J.S., Tipton, C.M., & Vailas, A.C. (1982). Exercise, physical training and the ageing process. In A. Viiduk (Ed.), *Lectures in gerontology, vol. 1B* (pp. 407-439). New York: Academic Press.

SMIDT, G.L. (1973). Biomechanical analysis of knee flexion and extension. *Journal of Biomechanics,* **6**, 79-92.

STEEN, B. (1988). Body composition in aging. *Nutrition Reviews,* **46**, 45-51.

THORSTENSSON, A., Grimby, G., & Karlsson, J. (1976). Force-velocity relations and fiber composition in human knee extensor muscles. *Journal of Applied Physiology, 40*, 12-16.

TOMONAGA, M. (1977). Histochemical and ultrastructural changes in senile human skeletal muscle. *Journal of the American Geriatrics Society, 25*, 125-131.

YOUNG, A., Stokes, M., & Crowe, M. (1984). Size and strength of the quadriceps muscles of old and young women. *European Journal of Clinical Investigation, 14*, 282-287.

YOUNG, A., Stokes, M., & Crowe, M. (1985). The size and strength of the quadriceps muscles of old and young men. *Clinical Psychology, 5*, 145-154.

Balance—To Stand or Fall

Helen M. Eckert
University of California–Berkeley

Although falls may be caused by factors other than balance per se, some aspect of the neuromuscular complex that enables an individual to maintain balance has been disturbed when a fall occurs. Recent investigations of the incidence of falls continue to support the observations of Sheldon (1950) that the number of falls increases with age and is proportionately higher for women. However, the death rate due to falls is higher for men than women at ages 75 and older (Ochs, Newberry, Lenhardt, & Harkins, 1985).

A sternal pressure test, in which only a slight sway of the body in response was considered normal whereas an abnormal response involved more movement, was used by Wild, Nayak, and Isaacs (1981) as a test of balance. Of the 38 fallers whose response was normal, only 2 died the following year, whereas 30 of the 77 subjects whose response was abnormal died in the same period. In addition, an age- and sex-matched study of 125 fallers and 125 controls over a 12-month period indicated that the number of deaths during this period was greater for the fallers than for the control group. The main factor associated with the increased mortality of the fallers was the impaired mobility in these persons aged 65 and older (Wild et al., 1981).

Concern about the increase of falls with increasing age, coupled with a higher death rate for fallers, generated a Symposium on Falls in the Elderly that included reviews of gait and balance (Wolfson, Whipple, Amerman, Kaplan, & Kleinberg, 1985), sensorimotor deficits related to postural stability (Stelmach & Worringham, 1985), and the implications for falls of spatial orientation mechanisms (Leibowitz & Shupert, 1985). The contents of these excellent surveys will not be duplicated here; rather, emphasis will be placed upon other recent observations of postural stability.

POSTURAL SWAY

Postural instability, or amount of sway as measured by a force plate, increases with age, and the increment is more in a one-foot stand with eyes open than in normal standing. Increases with age for anteroposterior sway during normal standing are somewhat greater than for lateral sway, and increments in both types of sway are greater for the eyes closed than the eyes open condition. Standing on one foot with eyes open results in marked increases in both directions of postural sway at all age levels, but especially for the 71- to 75-year-old men studied by

Era and Heikkinen (1985). These investigators found that postural sway behavior was correlated with percentage of body fat, aerobic and anaerobic capacity, grip strength, and vibratory threshold on the ankles within the three age groups examined.

Crilly et al. (1987) also report a greater lateral and anteroposterior sway in postmenopausal women who had suffered Colles' fracture in comparison with postmenopausal women without Colles' fracture. As the Colles' fracture subjects were not tested for sway until after they had recovered from the fracture, it cannot be assumed that they had the same degree of sway prior to the fracture. Reduction in mobility after a fracture or a fall may be a factor in increased sway, as Isaacs (1985) reports a reduced mobility index associated with increased sway path and reduced gait speed for 24 elderly people living at home. Similarly Mathias, Nayak, and Isaacs (1986) report an inverse relationship between sway path and gait speed for 32 elderly subjects with balance disturbances.

Sway, as measured by a force plate, has been shown by Visser (1983) to be greater in patients with senile dementia of Alzheimer's type (SDAT), as has lower gait speed. In comparison with normal controls, demented patients were also found to have significantly shorter step length, lower stepping frequency, greater step-to-step variability, and greater double support ratio. Observations of patients with senile dementia and of healthy aging subjects over a 50-month period have indicated that serious falls occurred in 36% of the SDAT individuals, as contrasted with only 11% of the controls (Morris, Rubin, Morris, & Mandel, 1987). Poor balance is also reported to be one of the characteristics associated with falls in patients with Alzheimer's type dementia (Buchner & Larson, 1987).

Although a previous report (Fernie, Gryfe, Holliday, & Llewellyn, 1982) of the relationship between postural sway in standing to incidence of falls in geriatric subjects concluded that there was a significant difference in mean speed of sway between fallers and nonfallers, the subsequent reanalysis of these data using a different statistical classification methodology pointed to a misclassification of both groups due to the overlap of their distributions (Bartlett, Maki, Fernie, Holliday, & Gryfe, 1986). The fact that the speed of sway does not appear, on the basis of reanalysis, to be highly predictive in categorizing fallers and nonfallers may be a feature of the test used to measure sway (movement of the pelvic girdle) as well as the sample distribution.

OTHER FACTORS

If sway alone is not a good predictor of the complex act of balancing, then perhaps this measure combined with muscle strength may prove predictive, as Buchner and Larson (1987) also list muscular weakness as one of the patient characteristics associated with falls in SDAT, and Tinetti (1987) reports that injured fallers were almost four times more likely to have lower extremity weakness than noninjured fallers. Whipple, Wolfson, and Amerman (1987) compared the strength of knees and ankles of a group of nursing home residents who had a history of falls with a group of age-matched controls. The results showed the nonfallers to be significantly greater in mean power and peak torque than the fallers in both knee and ankle musculature, with the ankle dorsiflexion power production in fallers being the most affected of all the motions tested. The difference in mean power between the fallers and nonfallers was greater at the higher limb velocities than at the lower limb velocities. As the ability of the body to recover balance often requires rapid movement to prevent a fall, the muscle strength difference, especially at the higher velocities, may be a crucial factor in maintaining balance.

A survey of a representative population of 425 women and 333 men, aged 75 years, indicated that the most common postural disturbances were a feeling of unsteadiness when rising from lying to standing, and when walking (Sixt & Ladahl, 1987). These activities require muscle strength in addition to the integrative functioning of the sensory modalities associated with balance. A postural stress test, which uses a pulley-weight system to deliver a reproducible impulse of destabilizing force to a subject, has been developed by Wolfson, Whipple, Amerman, and Kleinberg (1986) and administered to nursing home residents—both fallers and nonfallers—of equivalent age and sex as well as to younger controls. The results indicated significant differences between all three groups in balance strategy scores, with the fallers having consistently lower ranks than the nonfallers and the young subjects. As fallers had a bimodal distribution, with half recording the lowest scores and the other half clustering just below the old nonfallers, this test may be no more discriminatory of fallers and nonfallers in the same age group than the other tests of balance.

Increases in precision of force plates and of analytical potential in recording instrumentation may provide more discriminatory power to sway as a measure of balance (Hlavacka & Njiokiktjien, 1985; Tropp, Odenrick, Sandlund, & Odkvist, 1987; Yoneda & Tokumasu, 1986). However, balance is multifaceted, as pointed out in the review by Wolfson et al. (1985) and as indicated by studies such as the visual and vestibular contribution to pitch sway in the ankle muscles (Allum & Pfaltz, 1985) and of vertigo due to whiplash injury (Hinoki, 1985), which have attempted to elucidate the role of spinal reflexes associated with equilibrium. Complaints of instability have been found by Norre, Forrez, and Beckers (1987) to be increasingly associated with abnormal sway in older subjects, with compensation in elderly people being less efficacious at the vestibulo-spinal level than at the vestibulo-ocular reflex level. Clearly, the brain as well plays a crucial role in balance maintenance, and the increasing precision of positron emission tomography promises to make a considerable contribution to our understanding of the balance complex.

ACTIVITY EFFECTS

Although we do not have a complete understanding of the balance complex nor appear able to measure it accurately, it is becoming increasingly obvious that the individual's activity level, especially as one gets older, is closely associated with balance. For example, Rikli and Busch (1986) have found that 20 older women ($M=68.7$ years) who had participated in vigorous activity for the past 10 years or more on a regular basis had better balance, as measured by a one-foot stand, than did 20 inactive women of the same age grouping. Similarly, Vellas, Cayla, Bocquet, de Pemille, and Albarede (1987) report that the activity level of fallers, 65 years and older, was significantly less both before and after falls than for same-age and sex controls.

Improvements in balance performance have been reported by Roberts (1985) after a 6-week walking program in which the 72-year-olds walked for 30 minutes three times a week. In comparison with 30 age-matched controls, the 31 walkers improved significantly from pre- to posttest on the combined score of four stances whereas no change was reported for the control group. The effects of mental practice on balance in 70-year-old women have also been examined by Fansler, Poff, and Shepard (1985), who noted that the group that participated in the mental-practice-plus-physical-practice program had a significant pre/post improvement percentage in contrast to the nonsense-plus-physical-practice and the relaxation-plus-physical-practice groupings, which had nonsignificant pre/post improvement percentages. In this experiment, the intervention for each group consisted of prerecorded instructions with those of the mental facilitation group including suggestions for vivid visual images related to the one-legged balance task.

In summary, balance performance decreases with increasing age, especially after the sixth decade. However, the more active individual tends to maintain a higher performance level and a reduced degree of decrement. In addition, increased activity level, that is, practice, will improve performance and/or reduce the rate of decrement at all age levels.

> I am not confident when descending stairs. Recently I have felt I should carry a cane as many of my fellow residents do before they begin to use walkers. I have thought that my uneasiness is due to slow reaction—thought that perhaps nerve impulse was delayed for some reason—traveled slower in fiber?—slower in crossing synapse? A friend thought there was some relation to the ear. (Excerpt from a letter written by Ruth Glassow, age 96)

REFERENCES

ALLUM, J.H.J., & Pfaltz, C.R. (1985). Visual and vestibular contributions of pitch sway stabilization in the ankle muscles of normals and patients with bilateral peripheral vestibular deficits. *Experimental Brain Research,* **58,** 82-94.

BARTLETT, S.A., Maki, B.E., Fernie, G.R., Holliday, P.J., & Gryfe, C.I. (1986). On the classification of a geriatric subject as a faller or nonfaller. *Medical and Biological Engineering and Computing,* **24,** 219-222.

BUCHNER, D.M., & Larson, E.B. (1987). Falls and fractures in patients with Alzheimer-type dementia. *Journal of the American Medical Association,* **257,** 1492-1495.

CRILLY, R.G., Richardson, L.D., Roth, J.H., Vandervoort, A.A., Hayes, K.C., & Mackenzie, R.A. (1987). Postural stability and Colles' fracture. *Age and Ageing,* **16,** 133-138.

ERA, P., & Heikkinen, E. (1985). Postural sway during standing and unexpected disturbance of balance in random samples of men of different ages. *Journal of Gerontology,* **40,** 287-295.

FANSLER, C.L., Poff, C.L., & Shephard, K.F. (1985). Effects of mental practice on balance in elderly women. *Physical Therapy,* **65,** 1332-1337.

FERNIE, G.R., Gryfe, C.I., Holliday, P.J., & Llewellyn, A. (1982). The relationship of postural sway in standing to the incidence of falls in geriatric subjects. *Age and Ageing,* **11,** 11-16.

HINOKI, M. (1985). Vertigo due to whiplash injury: A neurological approach. *Acta Oto-Laryngologica,* **419**(suppl.), 9-29.

HLAVACKA, F., & Njiokiktjien, C. (1985). Postural responses evoked by sinusoidal galvanic stimulation of the labyrinth. *Acta Oto-Laryngologica,* **99,** 107-112.

ISAACS, B. (1985). Clinical and laboratory studies of falls in old people. Prospects for prevention. *Clinics in Geriatric Medicine,* **1,** 513-524.

LEIBOWITZ, H.W., & Shupert, C.L. (1985). Spatial orientation mechanisms and their implications for falls. *Clinics in Geriatric Medicine,* **1,** 571-580.

MATHIAS, S., Nayak, U.S.L., & Isaacs, B. (1986). Balance in elderly patients: The "Get-up and Go" Test. *Archives of Physical Medicine and Rehabilitation,* **67,** 387-389.

MORRIS, J.C., Rubin, E.H., Morris, E.J., & Mandel, S.A. (1987). Senile dementia of the Alzheimer's type: An important risk factor for serious falls. *Journal of Gerontology,* **42,** 412-417.

NORRE, M.E., Forrez, G., & Beckers, A. (1987). Posturography measuring instability of vestibular dysfunction in the elderly. *Age and Ageing,* **16,** 89-93.

OCHS, A.L., Newberry, J., Lenhardt, M.L., & Harkins, S.W. (1985). Neural and vestibular aging associated with falls. In J.E. Birren & K.W. Schaie (Eds.), *Handbook of the psychology of aging* (pp. 378-399). New York: Van Nostrand Reinhold.

RIKLI, R., & Busch, S. (1986). Motor performance of women as a function of age and physical activity level. *Journal of Gerontology,* **41,** 645-649.

ROBERTS, B.L. (1985). Walking improves balance, reduces falls. *American Journal of Nursing,* **85,** 1397.

SHELDON, J.H. (1950). Medical–social aspects of the aging process. In M. Derber (Ed.), *The aged and society.* Champaign, IL: Industrial Relations Research Association.

SIXT, E., & Landahl, S. (1987). Postural disturbances in a 75-year-old population: 1. Prevalence and functional consequences. *Age and Ageing,* **16,** 393-398.

STELMACH, G.E., & Worringham, C.J. (1985). Sensorimotor deficits related to postural stability. *Clinics in Geriatric Medicine,* **1,** 679-694.

TINETTI, M.E. (1987). Factors associated with serious injury during falls by ambulatory nursing home residents. *Journal of the American Geriatrics Society,* **35,** 655-648.

TROPP, H., Odenrick, P., Sandlund, B., & Odkvist, L.M. (1987). Stabilometry for studying postural control and compensation in vertigo of central and peripheral origin. *Electromyography and Clinical Neurophysiology,* **27,** 77-82.

VELLAS, B., Cayla, F., Bocquet, H., de Pemille, F., & Albarede, J.L. (1987). Prospective study of restriction of activity in old people after falls. *Age and Ageing,* **16,** 189-193.

VISSER, H. (1983). Gait and balance in senile dementia of Alzheimer's type. *Age and Ageing,* **12,** 296-301.

WHIPPLE, R.H., Wolfson, L.I., & Amerman, P.M. (1987). The relationship of knee and ankle weakness to falls in nursing home residents: An isokinetic study. *Journal of the American Geriatrics Society,* **35,** 13-20.

WILD, D., Nayak, U.S.L., & Isaacs, B. (1981). Prognosis of falls in old people at home. *Journal of Epidemiology and Community Health,* **35,** 200-204.

WOLFSON, L.I., Whipple, R., Amerman, P., Kaplan, J., & Kleinberg, A. (1985). Gait and balance in the elderly. *Clinics in Geriatric Medicine,* **1,** 649-659.

WOLFSON, L.I., Whipple, R., Amerman, P., & Kleinberg, A. (1986). Stressing the postural response. A quantitative method for testing balance. *Journal of the American Geriatrics Society,* **34,** 845-850.

YONEDA, S., & Tokumasu, K. (1986). Frequency analysis of body sway in upright posture. *Acta Oto-Laryngologica,* **102,** 87-92.

The Role of Physical Activity in the Life Quality of Older Adults

Bonnie G. Berger
Brooklyn College of the City University of New York

The graying of the American population has been a slow, progressive shift. In the United States, average life expectancy jumped from 47 to 73 years between 1900 and 1980 (Fries, 1980). The 65-and-older population grew twice as fast as the rest of the population during the last two decades. It is estimated that by the year 2000 the percentage of Americans over age 65 will be 12%. By the year 2030, 20% of all Americans will be over 65 (Collins, 1987).

Quality of life for this rapidly growing segment of the population can no longer be ignored without disastrous consequences. For example, the present system of Social Security is crumbling. Rising medical costs threaten the level of medical care provided to the elderly and highlight perplexing questions in the newly developed field of medical ethics. Costs of hospitalization and prolonged stays in nursing homes threaten to reduce some senior citizens to paupers. Growing old in the United States can be an unpleasant if not a terrifying prospect associated with illness, immobility, and impotence. The new vitality of people over 65, however, suggests that the aging process need not evoke images of gloom.

As illustrated throughout this paper, the grim vision of aging is rapidly changing to a more cheerful view based on the latest gerontology research. Exercise, along with good heredity, nutrition, and personal habits, can greatly enhance life quality of senior citizens. Of course, aging does not begin suddenly at age 65 or 70! Technically it begins at birth. An inherent linear decline in functional capacity begins at approximately 30 years of age (Jette & Branch, 1981). Fortunately, this decline can be modified substantially by exercise, weight control, and diet (Bortz, 1982; Shephard, 1986). As noted by Smith (1981), "Some of the current research suggests that *50% of the decline frequently attributed to physiological aging is, in reality, disuse atrophy* [italics added] resulting from inactivity in an industrialized world" (p. 16). Exercise and healthful dietary and living habits (a) decrease the physical burdens of aging, (b) enhance psychological and emotional well-being, and (c) increase the likelihood of living to one's full life expectancy (85+5 years) (Spirduso, 1986; Toufexis, 1988).

The aging process is not completely understood, due to complex interactions between physiological, psychological, and social factors. Because exercise affects all three, it is almost impossible to distinguish between decreases in physical abilities resulting from physical inactivity and those resulting from the aging

42

process itself. For example, following years of insufficient physical activity, people in their 30s, 40s, and 50s begin to notice a lack of physical endurance, decreased strength, increased body fat, and sagging muscles. The decline in physical ability can lead to a variety of psychological and social changes. Physical decline from a lack of exercise might result in the interpretation that one is aging and that intense exercise might be harmful to one's health, inappropriate for one's age, or both. As a result, the person incorporates the feeling of being old in his or her self-concept and participates even less in physical activity. A self-fulfilling prophecy begins: Decreased physical activity produces even greater changes in physical ability and body composition, and the cycle continues as the individual exercises even less. (See Figure 1 for the exercise–aging cycle.)

The adage "act your age" greatly deters adult participation in physical activity. People exercise less as they age because of the social–psychological process of age grading. The age grading of exercise tends to be learned by age 20 (Ostrow, Jones, & Spiker, 1981). Even preschool children have reported that exercise is less appropriate for older people (Ostrow, Keener, & Peery, 1986-87). Since the age grading of exercise is learned early in life, it is not surprising that adults who were 60 or older viewed physical exercise as increasingly inappropriate as the individual advanced in age from 20 to 40 to 60 and to 80 years (Ostrow & Dzewaltowski, 1986).

Contrasting with the tendency to exercise less with increasing age is the increased need to exercise as one ages. An individual in his or her 30s who does not exercise can rely only on innate physical ability to perform daily tasks. By

THE EXERCISE - AGING CYCLE

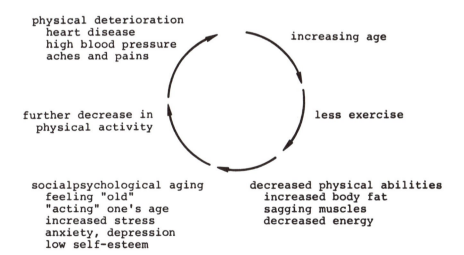

Figure 1 — The exercise–aging cycle. *Note.* From Berger & Hecht, "Exercise, aging, and psychological well-being: The mind-body question." In A.C. Ostrow (Ed.), *Aging and motor behavior* (in press). Indianapolis: Benchmark Press.

the time that person is 50 or 60, the lack of exercise has taken its toll. By exercising regularly, the elderly can increase their flexibility, muscle strength and endurance, aerobic capacity, balance, and agility (e.g., Shephard, 1986; Shephard & Sidney, 1979; Smith, 1981; Spirduso, 1986).

The relationship between physical functioning and psychological well-being at various stages of the adult lifespan is unclear (McPherson, 1986). Among the elderly, individuals who have good mental health tend to be physically active; physical activity is associated with enhanced mental health (Morgan & Goldston, 1987). Emphasizing the importance of psychological factors in the aging process, Pelletier (1981, p. 170) noted, "Psychological factors have been demonstrated to be the *single most significant predictor of both optimum health and longevity*" [italics added]. Such social–psychological factors play a key role in determining the amount of exercise pursued by adults throughout their lifespan.

PSYCHOLOGICAL HEALTH IN THE ELDERLY

The common perception that old people are cantankerous and crotchety is incorrect! There is considerable evidence that mental health tends to improve as one ages. Anxiety in particular tends to decrease with age. There is also some evidence that depression tends to be lower in people who are over 50 than in those between the ages of 19 and 49 (Lin, Ensel, & Dean, 1986). Although the elderly are no more depressed than other age groups, depression is the most common psychiatric complaint among the elderly (Gatz, Smyer, & Lawton, 1980; Rosenfeld, 1978). Depression in the elderly is difficult to treat because it often has real causes: failing health, loss of friends, and financial problems. Although the causes of depression in the elderly may differ from those in younger populations, there seems to be no relationship between age and outcome of therapy and/or the effectiveness of medication (Rosenfeld, 1978, p. 133). It is heartening to note that exercise is becoming an effective mode for treating depression in older adults (Bennett, Carmack, & Gardner, 1982; Martinsen, Medhus, & Sandvik, 1985; Morgan, Roberts, Brand, & Feinerman, 1970; Valliant & Asu, 1985).

A Developmental Perspective

When examining the mental health benefits of exercise for older adults, it is important to realize that adults in their 30s, 40s, 50s, 60s, 70s, and 80s are adjusting to very different issues (Helson & Moane, 1987; Levinson, Darrow, Klein, Levinson, & McKee, 1978). George Sheehan (1988), the noted sport philosopher and exerciser, aptly described some of the developmental changes in perception that occur in the aging process:

> To many people, growing old seems like the endgame in chess—life winding down in a series of small moves with less important pieces. As I age, I am discovering this is not true. . . . My life is not a defensive struggle of restricted options—*growing old is a game of verve, imagination, and excitement* [italics added].
>
> The aging game is chess at its best. . . . Some pieces have indeed been lost. But the board is still filled with opportunity. The outcome is not now a matter of strength, although that still remains, but of faith and courage,

hope and wisdom. . . . In the aging game I must be all I ever was and will be. What has gone before is no more than a learning period, a breaking in. Life, someone has said, is boot camp. If it is, aging is the combat for which I was trained. Now I must take the person I have become and make each new day special. I must make good on the promise of every dawn I am privileged to see. (p. 63)

Exercise definitely can play important roles in the developmental tasks of the elderly, as formulated by Havighurst (described by Schaie & Geiwitz, 1982). Developmental tasks of the elderly include the following:

1. Adjusting to decreasing strength and health—A regular program of exercise actually enhances muscle strength and decreases many age-related decrements! By exercising, older adults can increase their cardiorespiratory efficiency, decrease blood pressure, enhance muscular endurance, and retard osteoporosis (Berger & Hecht, in press; Rodeheffer et al., 1984; Smith & Gilligan, 1986).
2. Adopting and adapting social roles in a flexible way—The elderly can adopt new activities such as walking, swimming, and aerobics classes to replace the role of worker.
3. Establishing an explicit association with one's age group—Community organizations such as churches, age-group sport organizations, and senior citizens centers provide greatly needed opportunities to establish ties with other members of one's age group.
4. Adjusting to retirement and reduced income—It is critical that the retired individual replace work responsibilities with worthwhile, enjoyable activities. Exercise might be one such activity, especially for individuals who focus on accomplishment and productivity.
5. Adjusting to the death of a spouse—Losing one's life companion drains emotional resources. Since exercise has been associated with mood enhancement in older populations (e.g., Bennett et al., 1982; Long, 1983; Valliant & Asu, 1985), it may be helpful in returning to one's usual emotional state.
6. Developing satisfactory physical living arrangements—The elderly need easy access to shopping, medical care, friends, and recreational activities to avoid being a burden to their adult children (Schaie & Geiwitz, 1982). The individual who has developed and maintained his or her physical capacities has much greater flexibility in establishing preferred, workable living arrangements.

A Need for Caution

Highly disparate studies support the likelihood that physical activity in older people is associated with desirable personality characteristics, life satisfaction, mental health, and stress reduction (e.g., deVries & Adams, 1972; Hogan & Santomier, 1984; Morris, Lussier, Vaccaro, & Clarke, 1982; Young & Ismail, 1977, 1978). When reviewing such studies, however, it is important to acknowledge a multitude of methodological problems in the exercise and mental health literature. (See Berger, 1984, and Folkins & Sime, 1981, for a discussion of common problems.)

Randomly assigning participants to treatments and follow-up testing of the same individuals would greatly enhance the quality of the studies. Restricting the studies to those employing older subjects further limits the quality of available research.

Shephard and Sidney (1979) have described common biasing effects that tend to lead to "false positive" results in psychological studies of exercise. These biasing effects are particularly cumbersome in studies of the elderly: (a) attitudes reflected by program advertising and exercise leaders, (b) participants' desire to please investigators, (c) favorable attitudes to exercise prior to initiation of the study, and (d) medical and personal attention received during training and testing (Shephard & Sidney, 1979).

The Relationship Between Exercise and Personality in Older Adults

Personality, both by definition and as measured by objective tests, tends to be stable. Thus it should not be surprising that older people do not report personality changes after participating in exercise programs (e.g., Hartung & Farge, 1977; Young & Ismail, 1977, 1978). However, adults who exercise regularly tend to have more positive personality constellations than do the sedentary. Exercise programs designed to attract and retain physically active and sedentary senior citizens probably should differ in approach and focus, if not in the activities themselves.

The likelihood that adults who seek exercise might differ in personality from the physically inactive was highlighted in a study of fitness and mental health by Young and Ismail (1978). Men ($N=28$) between 21 and 61 years of age were divided into high- and low-fitness groups according to initial fitness levels. The volunteers then participated in a 4-month program of jogging, calisthenics, and recreational activities. When measured at both the beginning and end of the study, the high-fitness group was more imaginative (Factor M), adventurous (Factor H), and trustful (Factor L) than those in the low-fitness group, as indicated by their scores on the Personality Factor Questionnaire (16 PF) (Cattell, Eber, & Tatsuoka, 1970).

Supporting the more positive personality traits in middle-aged exercisers, highly fit individuals ($N=48$) reported more positive personality characteristics on the 16 PF than the general population (Hartung & Farge, 1977). The self-selected runners and joggers were between the ages of 40 and 60 years, exercised 3 days a week, and covered at least 2 miles. These men were significantly more intelligent (Factor B), imaginative (Factor M), self-sufficient (Factor Q_2), and forthright (Factor N) than the general population. They also were more reserved (Factor A), sober (Factor F), and shy (Factor H). Employing self-selected exercisers, many of whom had been running for 5 years, prohibited a causal interpretation of the personality differences.

Exercise and Life Satisfaction

Correlation between physical activity and life satisfaction is impressively high. Older people who are physically active tend to have more positive attitudes toward work, are in better health, report more stamina, and report greater ability to cope with stress and tension (Heinzelman & Bagley, 1970; Schaie & Geiwitz, 1982). Life satisfaction, in comparison to personality, does seem to change with exercise. In one study, men ($N=381$) between the ages of 45 and 59 were randomly assigned to either an exercise group that met three times a week for 18 months or to a control group (Heinzelman & Bagley, 1970). The exercisers reported significantly greater changes than the control group in (a) enhanced personal health (increased stamina, less stress, and more positive feelings about weight reduction), (b) increased work performance and more positive attitudes toward work, and (c) stronger exercise habits (increased walking and stair use, and decreased use of the automobile).

Happiness. Happiness, the focus of a study by Rosenberg (1986), would seem to be an important factor in overall life satisfaction. In older adults ($N=468$) there was a significant, positive relationship between the number of memberships in voluntary associations, regardless of type, and avowed happiness. The correlation between membership specifically in sport groups and happiness, however, was not significant. Older people in three different age groups (55–64, 65–74, and 75+) were no happier with a membership in a sports group than in a nonsport organization. Although it was not clear exactly what sports associations were, this finding was not surprising. Formal membership in sports organizations, especially at 65 years of age, may be quite different from being physically active. Avowed happiness and its relationship to exercise intensity, duration, and frequency for older adults is an important area of needed investigation.

Self-Efficacy. Another way that exercise may be associated with life satisfaction is by increasing self-efficacy. Self-efficacy, the belief that one is capable of performing a variety of tasks, denotes feelings of competency and power. People who are high in self-efficacy feel competent and thus attempt and persist in a wider variety of physical activities than those who are low in self-efficacy. Older people often underestimate their physical abilities because of the widespread ageism in American society (Hogan & Santomier, 1984).

In a study of the relationship between a 5-week swimming program and self-efficacy, older adults (age 60 or older) in the swimming class ($n=32$) reported significantly larger changes in swimming self-efficacy than did a nonswimming group of controls ($n=33$) (Hogan & Santomier, 1984). In addition, 78% of the swimmers reported generalized feelings of self-efficacy and competence. For example, one swimmer reported, "I am able to do things more easily now—swimming and chores" (p. 295).

Self-Concept, Self-Esteem, and Body Image. Exercise also might increase life satisfaction in the elderly by enhancing the participant's body image, self-concept, and self-esteem. In one of the few studies of body image and exercise in an older population, nursing home residents participated in rhythmic breathing, slow stretching, and upright exercises twice a week for 8 weeks (Olson, 1975). Their body image scores improved significantly. Sidney and Shephard (1976) also reported increases in body image scores for healthy volunteers (M age = 66) following an endurance program that met 4 days a week in 1-hour sessions for 14 weeks. This significant increase in body image did not occur in all participants; it occurred in those who attended the sessions regularly and exercised at a high level of intensity (pulse rates of 140–150).

Life Quality. This rather nebulous term refers to "the degree to which an individual is able to satisfy his or her perceived psychophysiologic needs" (Dalkey, Lewis, & Snyder, 1972). Life quality also refers to a state of excellence (Morris et al., 1982). A high level of life quality has been related to the extent of physical activity in college students and in masters age-group athletes (Morris & Husman, 1978; Morris et al., 1982). College students who participated in an endurance conditioning program reported a significant improvement in life quality (Morris & Husman, 1978). Women masters competitors (i.e., they were at least 40 years of age) who were nationally ranked were significantly higher in life quality than a normative group of nonrunning adults (Morris et al., 1982). Although there are no data concerning life quality and exercise in the elderly, it seems that life quality in this group would improve as the exercisers noticed and enjoyed the psychophysiological changes. A study at Brooklyn College is presently under way to test this possibility (Berger, Michielli, & Cohen, in preparation).

Exercise is Associated With Decreased Stress

Psychological stress occurs within the individual in response to events that excite, frighten, irritate, or confuse. Stress results from a person's negative appraisal of his or her ability to cope with a situation and causes a variety of psychological and physical responses (Berger, 1986). Too much stress is associated with increased illness and mortality rates (Benson, 1975; Levy, 1983; Maddi, Bartone, & Puccetti, 1987). It also detracts from the quality of life. The elderly are as prone to stress as are younger members of the population, if not more so. Common stressful events for this age group include retirement, decreased physical abilities, chronic illness, death of friends, financial problems, and undesirable changes in appearance.

Exercise is an ideal stress reduction technique for older adults because of its psychological and physiological benefits. It is accompanied by reductions in anxiety, depression, and anger—three common psychological stress symptoms (e.g., Berger, 1986; Morgan & Goldston, 1987; Sachs & Buffone, 1984). Exercise is also associated with improvement in participants' vigor and clear-mindedness or decisiveness (Berger & Owen, 1983, 1988). In addition, regular exercise reduces several physical symptoms of stress: elevated heart rate, blood pressure, obesity, and general muscular tension (deVries, 1981; Sharkey, 1984).

In comparison to other stress reduction techniques, exercise has specific advantages that are important to older individuals. The side effects of drugs are avoided and a variety of physical benefits accrue: weight reduction, enhanced cardiovascular endurance and energy, and improved appearance. Unlike biofeedback, it requires no expensive equipment (Berger, 1986).

Decreases in Muscular Tension and Self-Reported Anxiety. In one of the few studies of muscular tension and exercise in older adults, deVries and Adams (1972) investigated the tranquilizing effects of exercise. Men ($n=6$) and women ($n=4$) between the ages of 52 and 70 were recruited by advertisements for individuals who were nervous, tense, and under stress. Participants scored in the 87th percentile on the Taylor Manifest Anxiety Scale (Taylor, 1953) and served as their own controls in a double blind design. They were tested three times in each of the following treatments:

1. 15 minutes of walking at a heart rate of 100 beats per minute;
2. 15 minutes of walking at a heart rate of 120 beats per minute;

3. 400 mg meprobamate, a common tranquilizer;
4. placebo;
5. a control situation in which the subjects read (deVries & Adams, 1972).

Stress was measured by electromyographic recordings from the biceps. In this older age group, stress decreased significantly after the subjects walked at the heart rate of 100 beats per minute, but not at the rate of 120 beats per minute. Surprisingly, the meprobamate group did not report reductions in stress. The 400-mg meprobamate dosage, however, may have been too low to have been effective. Neither the placebo nor control groups reported any changes.

In another study of the effectiveness of exercise in reducing stress, Long (1983) compared the stress reduction benefits of a walk–jog program with those of stress inoculation (changing self-statements in anxiety-producing situations) and a wait list control group. The volunteers ($N=73$) felt they were unusually stressed and needed help to reduce their stress levels. They ranged in age from 24 to 65 years; mean age was 40. The women and men in both of the stress reduction programs met for 90 minutes once a week in supervised sessions for 10 weeks. In addition, they practiced one of the techniques independently twice a week.

Results of this study are particularly interesting because the study is one of the few to focus on exercise and the reduction of psychological stress in older individuals. Participants in both the walk–jog and stress inoculation programs reported significantly less tension, state anxiety, and trait anxiety at the end of the 10-week programs (see Figure 2). Since fitness improvement was not related to the benefits, Long concluded that the decreases in psychological stress seemed to be psychologically based.

Decreases in Depression, Another Stress Symptom. Exercise is associated with decreases in depression in older as well as younger individuals (Bennett et al., 1982; Martinsen et al., 1985; Uson & Larrosa, 1982; Valliant & Asu, 1985). One study, conducted in Spain, examined the effectiveness of exercise in adults between the ages of 60 and 80. Uson and Larrosa (1982) reported that 70% of those who exercised ($n=30$) for an hour twice a week for 9 months reported reductions in depression. The exercise program seemed to be of moderate intensity and included warm-up exercises, corrective gymnastic exercises, a 10-minute slow run, and psychomotor activities designed to improve coordination. In contrast to the exercisers, 40% of the age-matched controls ($n=30$) who belonged to clubs for retired persons experienced increased depression. The exercisers also reported fewer visits to the doctor than did the controls during the same 9-month period.

In another study, nursing home residents and participants at a senior community center ($N=38$) who were clinically depressed reported significantly less depression at the end of an 8-week exercise program (Bennett et al., 1982). The participants ranged from 50 to 98 years of age and exercised in 45-minute sessions twice a week. The relatively mild program included only balance and flexibility exercises.

Further supporting a relationship between exercise and decreased depression in older populations, psychiatric patients (ages 17–60, *M* age=40) indicated that they too were less depressed after exercise (Martinsen et al., 1985). In this well-

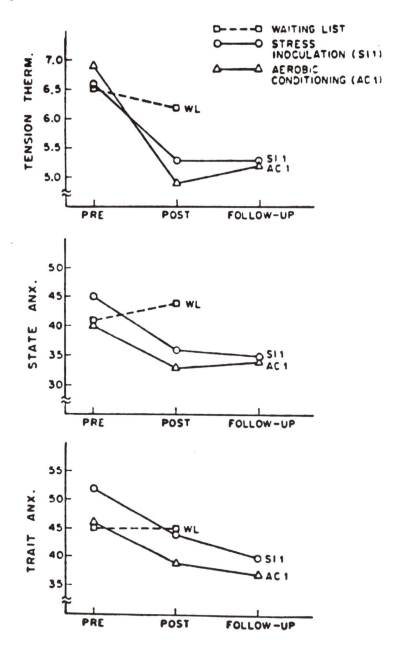

Figure 2 — Mean ratings of change on measures of stress before and after treatment, and at 3-month follow-up. *Note*. From "Aerobic conditioning and stress reduction: Participation or conditioning?" By B.C. Long, 1983, *Human Movement Science*, 2, 171-186.

designed study, depressed male and female psychiatric patients were assigned randomly to either an exercise ($n=24$) or occupational therapy control group ($n=19$). Initially the two groups did not differ in depression. Exercisers participated in supervised aerobic exercise at 50–70% of their maximum aerobic capacity three times a week. At the end of 9 weeks, the exercisers increased in aerobic capacity and decreased in depression. Among exercisers of all ages, a moderate intensity program is associated with antidepressive benefits.

EXERCISE GUIDELINES
TO ENHANCE THE PSYCHOLOGICAL BENEFITS

The relationship between exercise and quality of life in the elderly is complex, and some of the contributing factors probably have not yet been identified. Although many existing studies of older populations have major design inelegancies, it seems probable that the psychological benefits of exercise in the elderly are as large as those in younger populations. As reviewed in this paper, exercise has been associated with decreases in anxiety and depression, enhanced self-efficacy and life quality, and desirable personality characteristics.

Not *all* types of exercise are mood enhancing. In fact, competitive and/or exhausting exercise may be stress producing! To glean maximal psychological benefits, exercise programs should be tailored to the psychological needs and capabilities of various subgroups in the elderly. The most successful participants in physical activity are those who exercise in programs that set attainable performance goals (Ostrow, 1984). Unrealistic goal setting and over- or underestimation of performance ability cause frustration and can lead to failure. Competent exercise leaders who enjoy working with the elderly are crucial to program success. In addition, a sport psychologist associated with the program can help the elderly develop more positive attitudes toward physical capabilities and activity, decrease anxiety about exercise procedures, and improve their self-concept, self-efficacy, and the quality of life.

Enjoyment is a Critical Feature

Enjoyment is an important aspect of exercise programs designed to enhance psychological well-being (Berger & Owen, 1987; Wankel & Kreisel, 1985). Unpleasant environmental influences such as extreme heat and exercising too intensely can negate the stress reduction benefits (Berger & Owen, 1986, 1987, 1988).

Exercise Intensity

Aerobic exercise is frequently cited in the literature as a primary requirement for mood alteration (e.g., Goldwater & Collis, 1985; Long, 1983). However, there is little research directly investigating the relationship between exercise intensity and mood elevation. The psychological effects of mildly intense activities have been relatively neglected. In one study, deVries and Adams (1972) reported that exercising at a heart rate of 100 beats per minute did reduce muscle tension. However, Dishman (1986) concluded, "it appears that an exercise intensity exceeding *70% of VO_2 max or age-adjusted HR for at least 20 minutes* [italics added] is needed to insure an accurate reduction" in anxiety (p. 311). Exercise intensity exceeding 80% of maximal heart rate has not been associated with mood elevation (i.e., Berger & Owen, 1986, 1987, 1988). For the elderly, exercise intensity probably should be light (deVries, 1981; deVries & Adams, 1972) or moderate.

Comparing the mood benefits of swimming, body conditioning, Hatha yoga, and fencing, Berger and Owen (1988) reported that the college-age yoga participants in two different classes reported significant decreases in psychological stress. Although Hatha yoga does not result in aerobic benefits, participants reported less anxiety, tension, depression, anger, and confusion immediately after yoga sessions than before class on three different occasions (see Figure 3). Hatha yoga

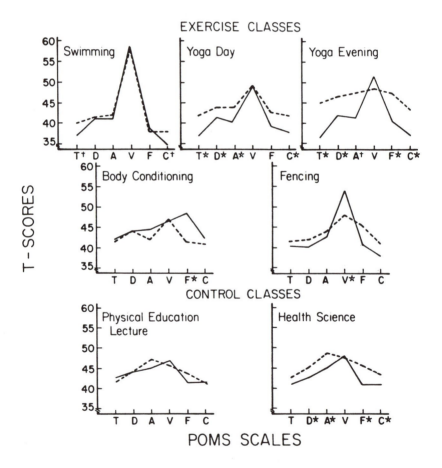

Figure 3 — Mean Profile of Mood States (POMS) *T* scores averaged across 3 days. Before-class scores are represented by a broken line; after-class scores, by a solid line. The POMS subscales include tension (T), depression (D), anger (A), vigor (V), fatigue (F), and confusion (C). ★ f < .05 on all 3 days; † f < .05 on 1 or 2 days. *Note.* From Berger & Owen, ''Stress reduction and mood enhancement in four exercise modes.'' In *Research Quarterly for Exercise and Sport, 59,* 148-159.

and many aerobic types of exercise facilitate rhythmical, abdominal breathing. Perhaps it is the rhythmical breathing rather than the aerobic quality that reduces stress.

Since the elderly are cautious about taxing their hearts with aerobic exercise, it is encouraging to note that aerobic exercise may not be a prerequisite for stress reduction. Although additional research on the relationship between exercise intensity and mental health is needed, it seems that older individuals can ease into exercise with a moderate program. They can reap some of the psychological benefits, condition their bodies, and gain confidence before initiating aerobic programs for cardiorespiratory conditioning.

Exercise Frequency

By exercising regularly, participants become progressively more fit and able to enjoy the physical exertion. Thus there is a need to exercise in the same activity at least twice, preferably three times, a week to enhance the mental health benefits (Berger, 1986; Glasser, 1976, p. 123). Habitual exercisers learn to pace themselves, to interpret various physical sensations, and to relax while exercising. These abilities are especially important for the elderly who may be unaccustomed to exercising. Another reason for the need to exercise regularly is that the psychological benefits are transitory in members of a psychologically normal population (Berger, 1987). Thus, most participants need to exercise frequently to retain the benefits.

Closed, Predictable Activities

Highly predictable or certain activities such as swimming, walking/jogging, and calisthenics have been described as "closed" (e.g., Berger, 1972; Singer & Gerson, 1981). One reason that self-paced, predictable physical activities are stress reducing might be that they enable participants to "tune out" or disassociate from the environment. Exercisers can engage in free association and can escape from daily stressors and hassles. This time-out opportunity may be especially beneficial to the elderly, who are besieged with seemingly insurmountable problems such as chronic illness, loneliness, and reduced incomes.

Absence of Interpersonal Competition

Since interpersonal competition tends to be stress producing, competition should be avoided if relaxation is a major goal. Glasser (1976) noted the importance of an absence of competition in his discussion of exercise and positive addiction. Positive addiction (PA), in direct contrast to negative addiction, leads to confidence, creativity, happiness, and health. As Glasser emphasized, "Not only must we not compete with others, we must learn not to compete with ourselves if we want to reach the PA state" (p. 57).

Duration: At Least 20–30 Minutes

Twenty minutes might seem a long time to exercise for many older persons. However, by beginning gradually, monitoring their target heart rates, and slowly increasing the duration, most healthy people in their 60s, 70s, and 80s can exercise for this length of time. In a study presently under way at Brooklyn College, several different groups of exercisers have increased their initial exercise sessions of 20 minutes to nearly 75 minutes (Berger et al., in preparation). The 20- to 30-minute session is a minimal amount of time suggested (Berger, 1986). Glasser (1976) and Mandell (1979) have suggested an hour or longer to maximize the psychological benefits.

CONCLUSIONS

Old age is no longer a time for only rest and disengagement. New role models are evolving, and the healthy elderly explore unchartered possibilities and challenge society's rules and norms. With the aid of a physically healthy lifestyle, an individual can be physically capable, energetic, and an exercise participant long beyond the ages of 50, 60, and 70!

Preliminary research data indicate that the psychosocial effects of exercise for older adults include a host of benefits. The elderly who are physically active report increases in life satisfaction, life quality, and happiness (e.g., Heinzelman & Bagley, 1970; Hogan & Santomier, 1984; Rosenberg, 1986). The elderly also report decreases in muscular tension and psychological stress indices, especially anxiety and depression (e.g., Bennett et al., 1982; deVries & Adams, 1972; Long, 1983; Martinsen et al., 1985; Uson & Larrosa, 1982; Valliant & Asu, 1985).

Despite the considerable need for additional research, there are enough data to suggest that exercise promotes psychological and physical well-being in the elderly. Organized exercise programs, individualized for the needs of specific subpopulations, are greatly needed to combat the ageism stereotypes that are rampant in American society. Diminished self-expectancies coupled with social expectancies that one should act his or her age greatly reduce the amount of exercise most older individuals pursue. Supervised exercise programs that encourage the elderly to explore, develop, and extend their physical capabilities are urgently needed.

Exercise programs that contain many of the following characteristics seem more conducive to mood alteration than those programs that contain less. To enhance the psychological benefits of exercise for the elderly, the supervised program should be enjoyable. In addition it should promote abdominal breathing and be noncompetitive. By exercising three times a week or more, the elderly can be comfortable with the moderate level of exercise intensity that seems to promote mood alteration. To maximize the likelihood of the psychological benefits, the older individual should participate at least 20 to 30 minutes a session.

A Look to the Future

Throughout this paper I have presented my beliefs as well as research data suggesting that exercise can enhance the quality of life in older individuals. It is hoped that the present review will encourage researchers to focus on the psychosocial aspects of exercise for the elderly. A few of the many topics that need specific attention are as follows:

- Refinement of exercise guidelines that promote mental health in older adults;
- Examination of the complex interrelationships between psychological stress, exercise, and the aging process;

- The therapeutic value of exercise in treating elderly patients who are anxious or depressed;
- The influence of exercise on self-concept, self-esteem, and body image in older adults;
- Exploration of mechanisms, physiological and psychological, that mediate the relationship between exercise and quality of life in senior citizens;
- Factors that promote exercise adherence in the elderly;
- Social–psychological benefits of exercise for the institutionalized old.

REFERENCES

BENNETT, J., Carmack, M.A., & Gardner, V.J. (1982). The effect of a program of physical exercise on depression in older adults. *Physical Educator, 39*, 21-24.

BENSON, H. (1975). *The relaxation response.* New York: Avon.

BERGER, B.G. (1972). Relationships between the environmental factors of temporal spatial uncertainty, probability of physical harm, and nature of competition and selected personality characteristics of athletes. *Dissertation Abstracts International, 33*, 1014A. (University Microfilms No. 72-23689, 373)

BERGER, B.G. (1984). Running away from anxiety and depression: A female as well as male race. In M.L. Sachs & G.W. Buffone (Eds.), *Running as therapy: An integrated approach* (pp. 138-171). Lincoln: University of Nebraska Press.

BERGER, B.G. (1986). Use of jogging and swimming as stress reduction techniques. In J.H. Humphrey (Ed.), *Current selected research in human stress* (Vol. 1, pp. 169-190). New York: AMS Press.

BERGER, B.G. (1987). Stress reduction following swimming. In W.P. Morgan & S.E. Goldston (Eds.), *Exercise and mental health* (pp. 139-143). Washington, DC: Hemisphere.

BERGER, B.G., & Hecht, L. (in press). Exercise, aging, and psychological well-being: The mind–body question. In A.C. Ostrow (Ed.), *Aging and motor behavior.* Indianapolis: Benchmark Press.

BERGER, B.G., Michielli, D., & Cohen, K. (in preparation). *Life quality and exercise in the elderly.*

BERGER, B.G., & Owen, D.R. (1983). Mood alteration with swimming—Swimmers really do "feel better." *Psychosomatic Medicine, 45*, 425-433.

BERGER, B.G., & Owen, D.R. (1986). Mood alteration with swimming: A re-evaluation. In L. Vander Velden & J.H. Humphrey (Eds.), *Current selected research in the psychology and sociology of sport* (Vol. 1, pp. 97-114). New York: AMS Press.

BERGER, B.G., & Owen, R.D. (1987, September). *Preliminary analysis of a causal relationship between swimming and anxiety: Fatigue may negate the psychological benefits.* Paper presented at the meeting of the Association for the Advancement of Applied Sport Psychology, Newport Beach, CA.

BERGER, B.G., & Owen, D.R. (1988). Stress reduction and mood enhancement in four exercise modes: Swimming, body conditioning, Hatha yoga, and fencing. *Research Quarterly for Exercise and Sport, 59*, 148-159.

BORTZ, W.M. (1982). Disuse and aging. *Journal of the American Medical Association, 248*, 1203-1208.

CATTELL, R.B., Eber, H.W., & Tatsuoka, M. (1970). Handbook for the Sixteen Personality Factor Questionnaire. In *Clinical education, industrial and research psychology.* Champaign, IL: Institute for Personality and Ability Testing.

COLLINS, G.L. (1987, April 2). As nation grays, a mighty advocate flexes its muscles. *The New York Times,* pp. C1, C8.

DALKEY, N.C., Lewis, R., & Snyder, D. (1972). *Studies of life quality.* Boston: D.C. Heath.

deVRIES, H.A. (1981). Tranquilizer effects of exercise: A critical review. *The Physician and Sportsmedicine,* **9**(11), 46-55.

deVRIES, H.A., & Adams, G.M. (1972). Electromyographic comparison of single doses of exercise and meprobamate as to effects on muscular relaxation. *American Journal of Physical Medicine,* **51**(3), 130-141.

DISHMAN, R.K. (1986). Mental health. In V. Seefeldt (Ed.), *Physical activity and well-being* (pp. 304-342). Reston, VA: AAHPERD.

FOLKINS, C.H., & Sime, W.E. (1981). Physical fitness training and mental health. *American Psychologist,* **36**, 373-389.

FRIES, J.F. (1980). Aging, natural death, and the compression of morbidity. *The New England Journal of Medicine,* **303**(3), 130-135.

GATZ, M., Smyer, M.A., & Lawton, M.P. (1980). The mental health system and the older adult. In L.W. Poon (Ed.), *Aging in the 1980s* (pp. 5-18). Washington, DC: American Psychological Association.

GLASSER, W. (1976). *Positive addiction.* New York: Harper & Row.

GOLDWATER, B.C., & Collis, M.L. (1985). Psychologic effects of cardiovascular conditioning: A controlled experiment. *Psychosomatic Medicine,* **47**, 174-181.

HARTUNG, G.H., & Farge, E.J. (1977). Personality and physiological traits in middle-aged runners and joggers. *Journal of Gerontology,* **32**, 541-548.

HEINZELMAN, F., & Bagley, R.W. (1970). Response to physical activity programs and their effects on health behavior. *Public Health Report,* **85**, 905-911.

HELSON, R., & Moane, G. (1987). Personality change in women from college to midlife. *Journal of Personality and Social Psychology,* **53**, 176-186.

HOGAN, P.I., & Santomier, J.P. (1984). Effect of mastering swimming skills on older adults' self-efficacy. *Research Quarterly for Exercise and Sport,* **55**, 294-296.

JETTE, A.M., & Branch, L.G. (1981). The Framingham disability study: II. Physical disability among the aging. *American Journal of Public Health,* **71**, 1211-1216.

LEVINSON, D., Darrow, C.M., Klein, E.B., Levinson, M.H., & McKee, B. (1978). *The seasons of a man's life.* New York: Knopf.

LEVY, S.M. (1983). Host differences in neoplastic risk: Behavioral and social contributions to disease. *Health Psychology,* **2**, 21-44.

LIN, N., Ensel, W.M., & Dean, A. (1986). The age structure and the stress process. In N. Lin, A. Dean, & W.M. Ensel (Eds.), *Social support, life events, and depression* (pp. 213-231). New York: Academic Press.

LONG, B.C. (1983). Aerobic conditioning and stress reduction: Participation or conditioning? *Human Movement Science,* **2**, 171-186.

MADDI, S.R., Bartone, P.T., & Puccetti, M.C. (1987). Stressful events are indeed a factor in physical illness: Reply to Schroeder and Costa (1984). *Journal of Personality and Social Psychology, 52*, 833-843.

MANDELL, A. (1979). The second second wind. *Psychiatric Annals, 9*, 57-69.

MARTINSEN, E.W., Medhus, A., & Sandvik, L. (1985). Effects of aerobic exercise on depression: A controlled study. *British Medical Journal, 291*, 109.

McPHERSON, B.D. (1986). Sport, health, well-being, and aging: Some conceptual and methodological issues and questions for sport scientists. In B.D. McPherson (Ed.), *Sport and aging* (pp. 3-23). Champaign, IL: Human Kinetics.

MORGAN, W.P., & Goldston, S.E. (1987). *Exercise and mental health.* Washington, DC: Hemisphere.

MORGAN, W.P., Roberts, J.A., Brand, F.R., & Feinerman, A.D. (1970). Psychological effect of chronic physical activity. *Medicine and Science in Sports, 2*, 213-217.

MORRIS, A.F., & Husman, B.F. (1978). Life quality changes following an endurance conditioning program. *American Corrective Therapy Journal, 32*, 3-6.

MORRIS, A.F., Lussier, L., Vaccaro, P., & Clarke, D.H. (1982). Life quality characteristics of national class women masters long distance runners. *Annals of Sports Medicine, 1*, 23-26.

OLSON, M.I. (1975). *The effects of physical activity on the body image of nursing home residents.* Unpublished master's thesis, Springfield College.

OSTROW, A.C. (1984). *Physical activity and the older adult: Psychological perspectives.* Princeton, NJ: Princeton Book Co.

OSTROW, A.C., & Dzewaltowski, D.A. (1986). Older adults' perceptions of physical activity participation based on age-role and sex-role appropriateness. *Research Quarterly for Exercise and Sport, 57*, 167-169.

OSTROW, A.C., Jones, D.C., & Spiker, D.D. (1981). Age role expectations and sex role expectations for selected sport activities. *Research Quarterly for Exercise and Sport, 52*, 216-227.

OSTROW, A.C., Keener, R.E., & Perry, S.A. (1986-1987). The age grading of physical activity among children. *International Journal of Aging and Human Development, 24*, 101-111.

PELLETIER, K.R. (1981). *Longevity: Fulfilling our biological potential.* New York: Dell.

RODEHEFFER, R.J., Gerstenblith, G., Becker, L.C., Fleg, J.L., Weisfeldt, M.L., & Lakatta, E.G. (1984). Exercise cardiac output is maintained with advancing age in healthy human subjects: Cardiac dilation and increased stroke volume compensate for a diminished heart rate. *Circulation, 69*, 203.

ROSENBERG, E. (1986). Sport voluntary association involvement and happiness among middle-aged and elderly Americans. In B. McPherson (Ed.), *Sport and aging* (pp. 45-52). Champaign, IL: Human Kinetics.

ROSENFELD, A.H. (1978). *New views on older lives: A sampler of NIMH-sponsored research and service programs* (DHEW Publication No. ADM 78-687). Washington, DC: U.S. Government Printing Office.

SACHS, M.L., & Buffone, G.W. (Eds.) (1984). *Running as therapy: An integrated approach.* Lincoln: University of Nebraska Press.

SCHAIE, K.W., & Geiwitz, J. (1982). *Adult development and aging.* Boston: Little, Brown.

SHARKEY, B.J. (1984). *Physiology of fitness* (2nd ed.). Champaign, IL: Human Kinetics.

SHEEHAN, G. (1988). Playing the aging game. *The Physician and Sportsmedicine,* **16**(3), 63.

SHEPHARD, R.J. (1986). Physical activity and aging in a post-industrial society. In B.D. McPherson (Ed.), *Sport and aging* (pp. 37-43). Champaign, IL: Human Kinetics.

SHEPHARD, R.J., & Sidney, K.H. (1979). Exercise and aging. In R. Hutton (Ed.), *Exercise and sport science reviews* (pp. 1-57). Philadelphia: Franklin Press.

SIDNEY, K.H., & Shephard, R.J. (1976). Attitudes toward health and physical activity in the elderly: Effects of a physical training program. *Medicine and Science in Sport,* **8**, 246-252.

SINGER, R.N., & Gerson, R.F. (1981). Task classification and strategy utilization in motor skills. *Research Quarterly for Exercise and Sport,* **52**, 100-112.

SMITH, E.L. (1981). Age: The interaction of nature and nurture. In E.L. Smith & R.C. Serfass (Eds.), *Exercise and aging: The scientific basis* (pp. 11-17). Hillside, NJ: Enslow.

SMITH, E.L., & Gilligan, C. (1986). Exercise, sport, and physical activity for the elderly: Principles and problems of programming. In B.D. McPherson (Ed.), *Sport and aging* (pp. 91-105). Champaign, IL: Human Kinetics.

SPIRDUSO, W.W. (1986). Physical activity and the prevention of premature aging. In V. Seefeldt (Ed.), *Physical activity and well-being* (pp. 142-160). Reston, VA: AAHPERD.

TAYLOR, J.A. (1953). A personality scale of manifest anxiety. *Journal of Abnormal and Social Psychology,* **48**, 285-290.

TOUFEXIS, A. (1988, February 22). Older—But coming on strong. *Time,* pp. 76-79.

USON, P.P., & Larrosa, V.R. (1982). Physical activities in retirement age. In J. Partington, T. Orlick, & J. Salmela (Eds.), *Sport in perspective* (pp. 149-151). Ottawa, Canada: Coaching Association of Canada.

VALLIANT, P.M., & Asu, M.E. (1985). Exercise and its effects on cognition and physiology in older adults. *Perceptual Motor Skills,* **61**, 1031-1038.

WANKEL, L., & Kreisel, P.S. (1985). Factors underlying enjoyment of youth sports: Sport and age group comparisons. *Journal of Sport Psychology,* **7**, 51-64.

YOUNG, J.R., & Ismail, A.H. (1977). Comparison of selected physiological and personality variables in regular and nonregular adult male exercisers. *Research Quarterly,* **48**, 617-622.

YOUNG, J.R., & Ismail, A.H. (1978). Ability of biochemical and personality variables in discriminating between high and low physical fitness levels. *Journal of Psychosomatic Research,* **22**, 193-199.

Acknowledgments

Adapted from "Exercise, Aging, and Psychological Well-Being" by S. Berger and L. Hecht. In A.C. Ostrow (Ed.), *Aging and Motor Behavior* (in press). Indianapolis: Benchmark Press.

Supported in part by a Professional-Staff Congress-Board of Higher Education Research Award from the City University of New York, No. 6-65166.

Aesthetics and Meaningfulness of Movement in the Older Adult

Muriel R. Sloan
University of Maryland

The program for last year's Academy Meeting was devoted to an evolutionary view of physical activity in early and modern populations, with particular attention to the involvement of motor skills in bipedal locomotion and the making and use of tools. This year the program is organized to provide us with an evolutionary view of a single human life span, with particular attention to its aging phase. Most significant, however, is the inclusion of the topic "Aesthetics and the Meaningfulness of Movement in the Older Adult," the topic that Seymour Kleinman and I agreed to attempt to address briefly as footnote and postscript.

Inclusion of this topic, in my view, shows a sensitivity to the need to re-examine and re-address the scope and breadth of our field's involvement with and contributions to the human movement experience. The words in the title—Aesthetics . . . Meaningfulness . . . Movement—open up (a) recognition of the language and communication aspects of movement, for the mover and for the observer of movement; (b) recognition of the body as an instrument of self-expression as well as an instrument for accomplishing things; (c) recognition that movement is more than the term *physical activity* connotes—that it is an integration or oneness of body and mind; and (d) recognition that the qualitative aspects of movement experience, whether in exercise, sports, dance, or in sweeping the floor, has meaning throughout the life span.

Here I would like to make some observations.[1] First, movement means more than getting from one place to another, more than exercising to increase cardiovascular capacity, more than scoring a point, more than winning applause on the dance stage or the athletic field. Perhaps other meanings of movement, uniquely basic to human development and experience, will have to receive renewed attention as we address the interests and the more limited capabilities of the older adult. Perhaps this renewed attention to movement experience for its aesthetic value, for self-identity and expressiveness, for lifelong satisfaction, will influence the experiences we encourage and provide at earlier ages. An example is the simple everyday act of bipedal locomotion—walking. The evolution of walking in the human progresses from clumsiness to growing neuromuscular efficiency (and decreasing attention) to a fully automated skill. For sheer pleasure or for exploration of their expanding world, children can "play with" their walking. They can create new ways of getting from one place to another; they can enjoy the process and sensations of walking, and of seeing things and thinking things as they do so. Do we help children to experience walking in these ways, as well as monitoring heart rate, steps per minute, and so on? If not, can we expect them to do so as older adults?

Second, aesthetic experience in dance and sports is most often associated with high skill and long training. Maslow's writing on peak experience (1964) is a frequently drawn analogy, particularly in sports. Beauty in movement is in the kinesthetic feedback relative to the intent and capability of the mover. Perhaps our aestheticians and philosophers can help us broaden this concept of aesthetic experience and can help us bring the opportunity for such experience to all people throughout the life span.

Third, many of the most successful movement and exercise programs for older adults focus on the rhythmic nature of the activity, using music or other accompaniment. Frankel and Richard (1977), for example, present mobility exercises for the older person. The authors cite the following centuries-old pronouncement by Plato as still relevant to present day populations.

> Now health in body and mind which controls and improves the body, is to be obtained through music and gymnastics, which should continue throughout life—and he who mingles music with gymnastics in the fairest proportions, and best attempters them to the soul, may be called the true harmonist in a far higher sense than the tunes of strings. (p. 8)

Fourth, Ruth B. Glassow at age 96 is a primary source. During her career she was a pioneer in the scientific analysis of movement and is a walker to this day,[2] although in much reduced amounts. I asked her what movement meant to her. At first she responded by referring to the body mechanisms for movement and the changes in the neuromuscular system that come with age. When I prompted her with the word "meaning," she said she had seldom moved just to move, without an outside purpose. She had never been able to understand what the joy was in "just" a movement. Long ago she attended a class of Marge H'Doubler's and one day "Had a feeling—kind of exhilarating!" Marge said to her, "You're getting it!" Ruth said, "I do not know what Marge saw but she was right." After more thought on the topic, she exclaimed that the human body is the most wonderful entity and it is a pleasure to keep this instrument for movement in good working order to experience the joy of moving skillfully. She also said that most of the women living in her retirement home, unfortunately, were not as interested in movement.

Fifth, "It can reasonably be said that aging, especially among the very old, is mostly a woman's problem, both in the developed and developing nations." This is a direct quote from the 1982 edition of Aging and Mental Health (Butler & Lewis, 1982, p. xiii). In a 1980 review in the *Journal of Gerontology*, Spirduso reports that "not much information is available regarding the psychomotor performance of aging women, probably because the population of women exercisers over the age of 60 is very small" (p. 855). Although these two statements do not support a correlation between exercise and longevity, at least among women, they raise a question about the role and meaningfulness of movement experience in the quality of life. Should we expect women at age 60 and over to find typical models of fitness and exercise programs any more attractive than they did when they were 16? It is well past time to review the messages learned by at least 50% of the population through our activity programs in the schools . . . even as we must try to be creative in developing movement programs to interest and sustain the older woman as well as the older man.

REFERENCES

BUTLER, R.N., & Lewis, M.I. (Eds.) (1982). *Aging and mental health* (3rd ed.). St. Louis: C.V. Mosby.

FRANKEL, L.J., & Richard, B.B. (1977). *Be alive as long as you live.* Charleston: Preventicare Publications.

MASLOW, A.H. (1964). *Religion, values and peak experiences.* New York: Viking Press.

SPIRDUSO, W.W. (1980). Physical fitness, aging, and psychomotor speed: A review. *Journal of Gerontology, 35,* 850-865.

---

[1]Slides were shown of Dancers of the Third Age, part of the Dance Exchange of Washington, DC, and of the Adult Health and Development Program at the University of Maryland.

[2]Ruth B. Glassow died at her home in Madison, Wisconsin, on August 26, 1988 at age 96.

Aging and a Changing View of the Body

Seymour Kleinman
Ohio State University

I want to begin by reading a short excerpt from E.L. Doctorow's 1984 novel, *"Lives of the Poets."*

> Where is that nimbleness I never had? Where is that mind and body harmonic, that dream life in which I thoughtfully chew my food and take little sips of spring water, and I move in the philosophically enlightened way and I breathe from the diaphragm, a totally realized being in a serenity of pacific emotion, insufferableness, without guilt, without shame, fulfilled in each moment of life and memory in loving anticipation as the leanest brownberry guru? I cannot even stand up straight without wincing.
>
> I don't smoke anymore, that's something, I've cut down on beer and know clean air when I smell it, I know to eat bran, and acerola rose hips, and that sugar is bad and salt is bad, and eggs and anything pickled, smoked, or cured. But it's too much—all over the city, everyone running, shopping, consulting, trying to get away from this white-bread life, in their running suits they run, with their vegetable juicers under their arms. I've got more important things to do. What I need is a master guide to the wisdom, an exclusive service in the ideal location of the world, say, where you give all your money and all you ever hoped to have, and in return you receive a generosity of beneficent hygienically balanced natural unradiated lifelight and you get to live and write a minimum 150 years, give or take a decade. (p. 82)

This wistful, wishful confession rings a bell, I think, for all of us. It demonstrates our struggle to come to grips with our aging selves. It's a reflection of our urge to continue to see ourselves as we were in our prime, and it reveals our anxiety about losing our edge, our control.

Many might consider the healthy response in this condition to be, "Don't give in or give up." We admire Dylan Thomas' admonition: "Do not go gently into the night, Rage, Rage . . ." Giving up or giving in is not only wrong, it's immoral. But this is precisely what Doctorow reveals—this willingness and desire to place ourselves in the hands of an omnipotent "master" who will, for a fee, take care of us so we can get on with the more important things. But it also reveals a conception of the way we see ourselves as persons and of the way we view our bodies. And this is what I should like to explore.

Doctorow epitomizes this notion and compulsion to keep the body healthy in order to free the mind. This is not a new idea. It's just a reiteration of Platonic and Cartesian dualism that pervades our culture and that continues to exert enormous influence on contemporary education. As a result, physical activity has come to be viewed as some lesser form of human behavior. But I don't have to be telling you this. We, who are involved in physical education, have spent our professional lives battling this prejudice.

Yet compare this distinction, which is constantly made between mind and body, with the point of view taken in the following passage written by an extraordinary woman, Therese Bertherat, in a 1977 book, *The Body Has its Reasons*:

> Our Body is our Self. We are what we appear to be. The way we appear is the way we are. But we don't want to admit it. We don't dare look at ourselves. We don't even know how to look at ourselves. We confuse the visible with the superficial. We're only interested in what we can not see. We even go so far as to be contemptuous of the body and of those who are interested in it. Without stopping to understand our form—our body—we rush to interpret our content: our psychological, sociological, historical structures. All our life we juggle words so that they'll reveal the reasons for our behavior. And what if we were to seek, through our sensations, the reasons of our body?
>
> Our body is our self. It is our only perceptible reality. It is not opposed to our intelligence, to our feelings, to our soul. It includes them and shelters them. By becoming aware of our body we give ourselves access to our entire being—for body and spirit, mental and physical, and even strength and weakness, represent not our duality but our unity. (p. xi)

Doctorow, in the previously quoted passage, seems to regard his writing, his art, as separate from and alien to his body. But his wish for a master guide, someone who will watch over him and watch out for him, is an illusion. His body *is* his self, and his writing is an expression of that self. We do not and cannot function as separate entities. Doctorow's writing is his body. Our lives are our bodies. And, in a sense, our lives are our art.

Not giving up or giving in to aging may be admirable, but it is not sufficient. Anger, rage, and resistance are not long-term solutions. There is evidence to indicate that the contrary is true:

> After researchers at Johns Hopkins reported that cancer patients who showed angry defiance, a "fighting spirit" tended to live longer than did those who were passive and "good", Doctor Sandra Levy began to follow a group of thirty-six women who had been diagnosed as having advanced breast cancer. After seven years, twenty-four of the thirty-six had died. To her surprise, Dr. Levy found that, after the first year, anger made no difference in survival. The only psychological factor that mattered for survival within seven years seemed to be a sense of joy with life. That a joyous state of mind should be so powerful a predictor of survival was completed unexpected. (Goleman, 1987, p. 59)

It seems that it is important to get past that stage of anger and defiance in order to derive qualitative value from our experiences. This must of necessity take us beyond the negative, competitive, not-giving-up level, to the positive, meaning-seeking engagement in all that we do. This calls for a program of awareness about ourselves as bodily beings in the world. It calls for an intelligent and mature attitude toward movement and its meaning to us as we grow older. It should not be an abdication nor should it be an attempt to recapture the past; or a rage against growing older, which so often seems to be the case as we witness the proliferation of master's competitions and championships. This pervasive compulsion to measure performance in quantitative terms, unfortunately, seems to be a reflection of this attitude.

There are alternatives to these outer-directed, goal-driven activities. There are natural methods and movement awareness techniques that do not belittle our intelligence.

> These movements originate from inside your body; they are not imposed from the outside. There is nothing mystical or mysterious about them. Their goal is not to have you escape from your body, but to avoid having your body continue to escape you, and your life with it. (Bertherat, 1977, pp. 11-12)

The experience of activity should become an increasingly qualitative one for us as we age. It should provide and enable us to reach a level of maturity, self-knowledge, and enlightenment to which the young can only aspire.

REFERENCES

BERTHERAT, T. (1977). *The body has its reasons.* New York: Pantheon Books.

DOCTOROW, E.L. (1984). *Lives of the poets.* New York: Random House.

GOLEMAN, D. (1987, September 27). The mind over the body. *The New York Times Magazine,* p. 59.

Rather than an apology to, this is an affirmation of Soren Kierkegaard. It is, most assuredly, a "concluding unscientific postscript."

Biological, Functional, and Chronological Age

James S. Skinner
Arizona State University

There have been many attempts to develop indices or profiles of biological and functional age based on the assessment of various physiological, psychological, and social factors. The main purpose of these attempts has been to develop theoretical models with which to better understand the aging process, as well as to determine whether these aging processes could be manipulated (Heikkinen, 1982).

Shock et al. (1984) suggest that aging is more the result of an interaction among many specific characteristics within a person than of a single process. He and his co-investigators at the Gerontology Research Center of the National Institute on Aging (GRC-NIA) feel that aging is such an individual phenomenon that it can be characterized only by repeated observations of the same person. Thus, the usefulness of the various indices has been questioned (Costa & McCrae, 1985), and there is not much support for a "general process of aging" that controls all the physiological, psychological, and social aspects within an individual or a group of individuals.

EFFECTS OF AGING

The usual concept of aging is that the capacity of many functional systems within the body decreases over time. While aging is generally characterized by a decreased sensitivity and responsiveness to displacing stimuli (Skinner, 1987), there is no uniform pattern for all variables. According to Rockstein and Sussman (1979), for example, the rate of aging is not the same for all organs in any one organism or for any one organ among different individuals. Thus, aging is a progressive and irreversible process that occurs in everyone, but at different rates. Researchers at GRC-NIA (Shock et al., 1984) have identified the following six types of change:

1. Those functions that are stable or do not change with age (e.g., personality and resting heart rate);
2. Those changes related to illnesses associated with age, rather than to age itself (e.g., a drop in plasma testosterone does not occur in healthy men);
3. Those changes intrinsic to aging, that is, there is a functional decline despite the absence of disease (e.g., creatinine clearance drops in all);

4. Those changes occurring precipitously with old age. These are often secondary to or associated with disease (e.g., dementia);
5. Those secular changes that occur with time and have little or nothing to do with age or disease, probably reflecting cultural changes (e.g., a drop in serum cholesterol with age might be due to changes in eating habits and/or the availability of different kinds of food); and
6. Those changes that are compensatory (e.g., the Frank-Starling mechanism assists in maintaining cardiac output during exercise). People may also compensate by exercising regularly or stopping smoking.

What makes the concept of various types of profiles or indices even more complex is that what may be considered normal age-related changes in one country might be classified abnormal in another. For example, Skrobak-Kaczynski and Andersen (1975) found that the average percentage of body fat in a cross section of very active male Norwegian lumberjacks remained stable (14–15%) over the ages of 20 to 70 years. By comparison, the average values of American males increased from 12% to 25% over the same age span. In other words, people in many industrialized countries tend to be less active with advancing age, and this inactivity is often perceived to be natural (Skinner, 1987). Bourlière and Vallery-Masson (1985) also found differences in the aging process between urban and rural areas in industrialized countries.

CHRONOLOGICAL, BIOLOGICAL, AND FUNCTIONAL AGE

Chronological age is based on calendar time in years and is the only age that can be easily and accurately measured. There are many problems using only chronological age, however, because of differences in physical and mental function. For example, arbitrarily setting 65 years as the age of retirement was based more on economic and administrative reasons than on valid biological criteria (Heikkinen, 1982).

There appears to be no adequate definition of biological age. Because of the differences in the quantity and quality of any remaining function, there tends to be more variation in these functions as people age. While Heikkinen (1982) suggests that those who deteriorate least with age (i.e., are more stable) are biologically more youthful, the choice of biological properties to measure is critical, especially given the different patterns of change seen by Shock et al. (1984).

Assessing functional status seems to be a more rational basis for categorizing a person's age than is chronological age alone. Therefore, functional age is an abstract concept that makes logical sense, even if it is not easy to define or measure. Shock et al. (1984, p. 207) emphasize the need to consider "the interacting influences of biological processes, personality and behavioral factors, social and environmental forces, and the idiosyncratic health behaviors and stresses of the individual."

Instead of hypothesizing a single aging process, therefore, it is generally agreed that the best index of functional age is one that attempts to describe total functional status by combining results from physiological, psychological, and social factors that correlate highly with chronological age (Heikkinen, 1982). It is assumed that these factors describe the normal aging patterns.

INDICES OF FUNCTIONAL AGE

These indices are often devised by biometricians who make theoretical models of the mechanisms of aging (Comfort, 1979). After age-standardized norms for many variables have been statistically defined, simple linear and polynomial regressions with these variables versus chronological age as the dependent variable are used to determine a coefficient or weighting for each. The coefficients of those variables most closely related to chronological age are then combined into a single estimate or index. The assumption is that the average functional age calculated for a group of subjects will be close to its average chronological age. While the average functional and chronological ages of these indices may be similar, they are often criticized because of the large errors of estimate that are found. For example, Fozard (1972) derived a regression equation to predict age from a general aptitude test and had an error of 7.2 years.

Many test batteries for measuring rates of aging have been developed (e.g., Heikkinen, Kiiskinen, Käyhty, Rimpelä, & Vuori, 1974; Ries, Sauer, Pöthing, & Schwerdtner, 1976). Hollingsworth, Hashizume, and Jablon (1965) developed an index of physiological age using 437 Japanese men and women ages 10–70 years. They then used this index to study residents of Hiroshima exposed to radiation from the atomic bomb and found that radiation did not seem to affect aging. Dirken (1972) found a correlation coefficient of 0.87 between functional age scores and chronological age among 316 male Dutch industrial workers.

A major problem associated with these indices is their practicality, in that many test variables are included, requiring a great deal of time, personnel, and equipment to collect data. Another criticism raised by Shock et al. (1984) concerns the validity of these indices, that is, there has been no analysis to determine whether or not subjects whose physiological age was lower than their chronological age actually lived longer.

Perhaps the biggest criticism of these indices relates to their cross-sectional nature, that is, they try to determine normal aging patterns by looking at people of different ages and do not consider the possible longitudinal changes within people of the same age. In other words, cross-sectional data may give false impressions. Shock (1972) reported data on height and weight obtained from 470 men tested at least three times over 8 years. Although the average decrement in height in these men was similar to that seen with cross-sectional analyses, the same was not true for weight. Cross-sectional studies suggested that weight drops gradually from age 25 to 80 years. Longitudinal data, on the other hand, showed that men age 50 years and under gained weight, while those 55 and older lost weight. Shock et al. (1984) later suggested that accurate evaluations of longitudinal changes based on only three evaluations were too variable and unreliable. Similarly, Rowe, Andres, Tobin, Norris, and Shock (1976) did a longitudinal study on renal function and concluded that at least 18 years of observations were needed before one could accurately characterize the age-related changes in creatinine clearance within any one individual

In spite of these criticisms and problems, there are advantages to proposing and studying indices of functional age. They contain objective measures that can provide a better understanding of the aging process, and they are a fertile ground for generating and testing hypotheses on aging. It is also possible that one could modify the aging process by making changes in one's environment and lifestyle. Nevertheless, Shock et al. (1984) conclude that chronological age is not a reliable predictor of performance within an individual and that predictions based on physiological indices of aging are no better. Thus, it appears that this is a controversial area of research that can be justified on theoretical grounds when applied cross-sectionally to large groups, but is difficult to apply when attempting to explain the age-related changes within an individual over time.

REFERENCES

BOURLIÈRE, F., & Vallery-Masson, J. (1985). Epidemiology and ecology of aging. In J.C. Brocklehurst (Ed.), *Textbook of geriatric medicine and gerontology* (3rd ed., pp. 3-28). Edinburgh: Churchill Livingstone.

COMFORT, A. (1979). *The biology of senescence* (3rd ed.). New York: Elsevier.

COSTA, P.T., Jr., & McCrae, R.R. (1985). Concepts of functional or biological age: A critical review. In R. Andres, E.L. Bierman, & W.R. Hazzard (Eds.), *Principles of geriatric medicine* (pp. 30-37). New York: McGraw-Hill.

DIRKEN, J.M. (1972). *Functional age in industrial workers.* Groningen, Netherlands: Wolter-Noordhoff.

FOZARD, J.L. (1972). Predicting age in the adult years from psychological assessments of abilities and personality. *Aging & Human Development, 3,* 175-182.

HEIKKINEN, E. (1982). Assessment of functional ageing. In A. Viidik (Ed.), *Lectures on gerontology, Vol. IB* (pp. 481-516). London: Academic Press.

HEIKKINEN, E., Kiiskinen, A., Käyhty, B., Rimpelä, M., & Vuori, I. (1974). Assessment of biological age. Methodological study in two Finnish populations. *Gerontologia, 20,* 33-43.

HOLLINGSWORTH, J.W., Hashizume, A., & Jablon, S. (1965). Correlations between tests of aging in Hiroshima subjects. An attempt to define "physiologic age." *Yale Journal of Biology and Medicine, 38,* 11-26.

RIES, W., Sauer, I., Pöthing, D., & Schwerdtner, U. (1976). Methodische Probleme bei der Ermittlung des biologischen Alters [Methodological problems in the determination of biological age]. *Zeitschrift für die Gesamte Innere Medizin, 31,* 109-113.

ROCKSTEIN, M., & Sussman, M. (1979). *Biology of aging.* Belmont, CA: Wadsworth.

ROWE, J.W., Andres, R., Tobin, J.D., Norris, A.H., & Shock, N.W. (1976). The effect of age on creatinine clearance in men: A cross-sectional and longitudinal study. *Journal of Gerontology, 31,* 155-163.

SHOCK, N.W. (1972). Energy metabolism, caloric intake and physical activity of the aging. In L.A. Carlson (Ed.), *Nutrition in old age* (pp. 372-383). Uppsala, Sweden: Almqvist & Wiksell.

SHOCK, N.W., Greulich, R.C., Andres, R., Arenberg, D., Costa, P.T., Jr., Lakatta, E.G., & Tobin, J.D. (1984). *Normal human aging. The Baltimore longitudinal study of aging* (NIH Publication No. 84-2450). Washington, DC: U.S. Government Printing Office.

SKINNER, J.S. (1987). Importance of aging for exercise testing and exercise prescription. In J.S. Skinner (Ed.), *Exercise testing and exercise prescription for special cases* (pp. 67-76). Philadelphia: Lea & Febiger.

SKROBAK-KACZYNSKI, J., & Andersen, K.L. (1975). The effect of a high level of habitual physical activity in the regulation of fatness during aging. *International Archives of Occupational and Environmental Health, 36,* 41-46.

Physical Activity and Central Nervous System Integrity

Priscilla Gilliam MacRae
Pepperdine University

One of the most conspicuous phenomena associated with aging is the inevitable deterioration in physiological function that results in death. Biological age has been defined as "the process of change in the organism, which over time lowers the probability of survival and reduces the physiological capacity for self-regulation, repair, and adaptation to environmental demands" (Birren & Zarit, 1984, p. 9). Aging processes are characterized as inevitable, cumulative, and irreversible. The fact that physiological functioning declines with age is not questioned. However, rate of aging varies among individuals, and within each individual, body systems may decline at different rates. Thus it is evident that chronological age is not the best predictor of physiological functioning. In addition, it is suggested that certain aspects of the aging process can be modified by lifestyle choices such as physical activity.

The central nervous system (CNS), which includes the brain and spinal cord, is the principal regulatory system of the body. *Integrity* of the central nervous system refers to an unimpaired or unmarred condition of the brain and spinal cord. It is evident that the CNS controls the physical activities of the organism; however, the effects of physical activity on CNS integrity, particularly in the older organism, have been studied only recently. This chapter will discuss the effects of physical activity on the integrity of the aging CNS (see Figure 1). A brief review of the effects of age on physiological and behavioral functioning of the CNS will be included, followed by a discussion of the effects of physical activity on CNS integrity in young and old organisms. Mechanisms that possibly explain the physical activity effects on the integrity of the CNS of older organisms will be suggested in the final section.

AGING EFFECTS ON THE CNS: PHYSIOLOGICAL AND BEHAVIOR FUNCTIONING

Like most systems in the body, the CNS undergoes significant degeneration with old age. One of the first mechanisms to be investigated as an explanation of age-related behavioral decline was a change in cerebral circulation and energy metabolism. A multidisciplinary study carried out at the National Institute of Mental Health reported that cerebral blood flow remained stable in normal, healthy older adults for whom health and disease status was well controlled. However, researchers in this study also reported that the elderly subjects with evidence of

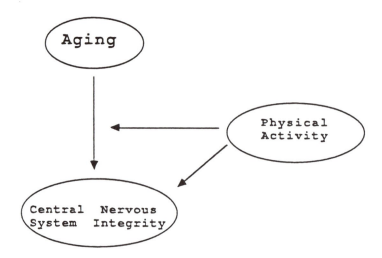

Figure 1 — Hypothesized relationships between aging, physical activity, and central nervous system integrity.

arteriosclerosis—even though minimal and asymptomatic—had significantly reduced cerebral blood flow compared with the young controls (Dastur et al., 1963). Cerebral glucose utilization, on the other hand, has been found to decrease in brain structures associated with vision, audition, and sensorimotor function even in healthy older adults (Dastur et al., 1963; Smith, 1984; Smith, Goochee, Rapport, & Sokoloff, 1980).

Age-related morphological changes, which include degeneration of cells in specific brain areas such as the locus coeruleus, substantia nigra, cerebellum, putamen, and cortex, also occur (Buell & Coleman, 1979; Peng & Lee, 1979; Scheibel, Lindsay, Tomiyasu, & Scheibel, 1975, 1976; Scheibel, Tomiyasu, & Scheibel, 1977; Vijayashanker & Brody, 1979). In addition, aging is associated with changes in the functions of various brain neurotransmitter systems. The catecholamine systems, particularly the nigrostriatal dopamine system, are most vulnerable to the aging process (Finch, 1976; McGeer, McGeer, & Suzuki, 1977; Samorajski, 1977). Many parameters such as striatal dopamine content, synthesis, turnover, uptake, and receptor binding are reduced in senescent rodents (Bhaskaran & Radha, 1983; Finch, Randall, & Marshall, 1981; Severson & Finch, 1980). Finally, disturbances in EEG patterns have been associated with the aging process (Wang & Busse, 1969; Wang, Obrist, & Busse, 1970). A detailed discussion of these topics can be found in *The Handbook of the Biology of Aging* (Finch & Schneider, 1985).

Since it is commonly accepted that the primary function of the CNS involves the regulation and control of behavior, it seems reasonable to assume that specific alterations in the physiological functioning of the CNS should be manifested ultimately in particular behavioral deficits. Much attention has focused on differentiating between behavioral functions impaired by aging and those functions spared from the effects of age. The most consistent behavioral change associated with the aging process is a slowing in speed of response, as measured by reaction time and movement time tasks (Birren, Woods, & Williams, 1979). The fact that speed of response is reduced with increased age is not only an acknowledged laboratory result but also of considerable practical importance (Salthouse, 1985).

Rapid responses are needed to prevent falls, to operate motor vehicles, and to function adequately in many daily living tasks. In addition to the practical importance of rapid motor responses, reaction time tasks are used to analyze cognitive processes of older organisms. It has been suggested that reaction time is one of the best behavioral measures of CNS integrity currently available (Birren et al., 1979). Age-related changes in other behavioral functions such as memory and cognition, mood parameters such as depression and anxiety, and personality variables such as self-concept and self-efficacy are discussed in detail in *The Handbook of the Psychology of Aging* (Birren & Schaie, 1985). It is important to note that investigators in the psychology of aging emphasize the interactional effects of environment factors, task demands, and health on the behavioral functioning of older adults.

PHYSICAL ACTIVITY EFFECTS
ON CENTRAL NERVOUS SYSTEM INTEGRITY

Physical activity has been defined in a variety of ways, but for this chapter physical activity will be defined as ''movement produced by skeletal muscles that results in energy expenditure'' (Powell & Paffenbarger, 1985). The evidence that chronic physical activity affects physiological and behavioral aspects of CNS function has been the focus of several studies over the past 10 years. Gilliam and her colleagues (1984) examined the effects of 3 months of daily running on dopamine receptor binding in young rats. Training effects were documented by an increase in cytochrome oxidase activity of the gastrocnemius/plantaris muscle of the running group. Dopamine receptor binding was measured by a dopamine agonist, spiperone. The running group had dopamine receptor binding values that were significantly greater than those of the control group (89 ± 13 vs. 60 ± 5 fmoles/mg protein). Other more recent studies have documented these results (DeCastro & Duncan, 1985; MacRae, Spirduso, Cartee, Farrar, & Wilcox, 1987).

Other neurotransmitters, norepinephrine and serotonin, have been shown to increase in response to chronic physical activity (Brown et al., 1979; Brown & Van Huss, 1973). Brown and Van Huss (1973) reported an increase in norepinephrine concentrations in the brains of trained rats when compared to sedentary rats. The exercise program was an 8-week interval-training treadmill protocol. The researchers expanded their results by examining norepinephrine and serotonin concentrations in three brain areas of young rats (the cerebral cortex, cerebellum, and remainder of the brain) following 8 weeks of treadmill exercise (Brown et al., 1979). The exercise consisted of 30 minutes of running, 5 days per week for 8 weeks. The researchers reported significantly greater norepinephrine and serotonin levels in most of the brain areas of the exercised rats when compared to the sedentary rats.

Cerebral blood flow during exercise has been examined in both animals and humans with differing results. Herholz and his colleagues (1987) reported an increase in regional cerebral blood flow of healthy young males during supine bicycle ergometer exercise at each of two different work loads, 25 and 100 watts. All six regions examined (frontal, parietal, temporal, occipital, precentral, and postcentral) showed significant increases in blood flow during exercise. The 12 subjects were randomly divided into two groups of 6 each with work load levels of 100 watts and 25 watts, respectively. The increase in cerebral blood flow in the 100-watt group (24.7%) was significantly greater than in the 25-watt group (13.5%). Increases in regional cerebral blood flow of exercising dogs has also been reported (Gross, Marcus, & Heistad, 1980). The regions of the brain that showed the greatest increase were those areas associated with motor function such as the motor-sensory cortex, cerebellar cortex, and spinal cord. Though these studies support *regional* cerebral blood flow changes with exercise, changes in *global* cerebral blood flow during exercise in humans and animals have not been found (Foreman, Snaders, & Bloor, 1976; Globus et al., 1983; Gross et al., 1980; Kleinerman & Sancetta, 1955; Pannier & Leusen, 1977; Zobl, Talmers, Christensen, & Baer, 1965).

The effects of habitual physical activity on behavioral functioning of young adults have been measured by examining such variables as cognition, mood, and personality. Hughes (1984) reviewed more than 1,100 articles on this topic and found only 12 articles that were randomized, controlled experiments with at least 10 subjects. These controlled experiments verified that exercise improves self-concept but do not indicate that exercise relieves anxiety or depression, or improves body image, personality, or cognition (Hughes, 1984). These results were corroborated by Tomporowski and Ellis (1986) in their review of published research on the effects of exercise on cognitive functioning. They concluded that the data obtained from studies failed to provide clear support for the notion that physical activity significantly influences cognition.

Few experimentally controlled studies have examined the effects of habitual physical activity on the behavioral functioning of the older adult (see Spirduso, 1983, 1984 for reviews). Cross-sectional studies provide substantial evidence that response speed, as measured by reaction time and movement time, is faster in older adults who maintain a physically active lifestyle, when compared to healthy but sedentary older adults (Clarkson, 1978; Rikli & Busch, 1986; Spirduso, 1975, 1980; Spirduso & Clifford, 1978; Spirduso, MacRae, MacRae, Prewitt, & Osborne, 1988). However, a few longitudinal studies have investigated the effects of an exercise program on the behavioral functioning of the older organism (Dustman et al., 1984; Samorajski et al., 1985). Dustman and his co-workers (1984) examined the effects of a 4-month exercise program (walk/jog) on neuropsychological function in older (55- to 70-year-old) sedentary individuals. Aerobically trained subjects were compared with two age-matched control groups: an exercise-control group that trained with strength and flexibility exercises and a control group that did not participate in supervised exercise. At the conclusion of the 4 months of exercise training, the aerobic exercise group had significantly higher maximal oxygen uptake ($\dot{V}O_2$max) than either of the control groups. The aerobic exercise group increased its $\dot{V}O_2$max by 27%, whereas the exercise control group increased its $\dot{V}O_2$max by 9%.

The aerobically trained group demonstrated significantly greater improvement on most of the neuropsychological measures (Critical Flicker Fusion, Digit Symbol, Dots Estimation, Simple Reaction Time, and Stroop tests). Sensory thresholds, indices of depression, and choice reaction times did not change significantly from initial values in any of the three groups. It appears that aerobic exercise training in previously sedentary older individuals can improve neuropsychological functions, which involve response time, visual organization, memory, and mental flexibility. The mechanism by which chronic physical activity affects behavioral function is unclear, but this topic has been the focus of recent studies.

It should not be surprising that neuropsychological function can be improved, because studies have documented that the "old brain" can be modified. Conner and colleagues have found that old rats who were housed in an environment that provided increased sensory and motor stimulation, which enhanced the size and complexity of neural structures, had larger and heavier forebrains and had enhanced cholinergic activity (Conner, Beban, Hopper, Hansen, & Diamond, 1982; Conner & Diamond, 1982; Conner, Wang, & Diamond, 1982).

Samorajski et al. (1985) examined the effects of voluntary wheel running exercise on various physiological and behavioral measures in C57B1/6J mice. The exercise was not introduced until the rats reached maturity (10–14 months). No significant differences in lifespan were found between the control group and the exercise group. However, it was found that exercise over the lifespan improved performance on the passive-avoidance test of recent memory. The positive effect of exercise on recent memory was greatest in the middle-aged rats (20–24 months old) but was also found in the old rats (28–30 months old).

In addition to the studies that explored the longitudinal effects of chronic exercise on behavioral aspects of CNS functioning in the older organism, a recent study examined exercise effects on physiological functioning of the aging brain. MacRae, Spirduso, Walters, Farrar, and Wilcox (1987) examined the endurance-training effects on aspects of dopamine function in the striatum of older rats. Male Sprague-Dawley rats (18 months old) were divided into a control group and a running group. The running group underwent a progressive 5-day-per-week exercise program for 3 months until the rats were able to run at a speed of 20 meters per minute for 60 minutes a day.

At 21 months of age both groups of animals were sacrificed along with a group of younger animals (6 months old). Citrate synthase activity of the gastronemius muscle was measured to document the endurance-training effects. The older running group showed a 27% increase in citrate synthase activity when compared with the older control group. Dopamine function in the brain's nigrostriatal system was studied by examining the relationship between the affinity and density of striatal D2 dopamine receptors versus steady-state levels of dopamine and its metabolites in the striatum. The results indicated that the older running group had a greater number of striatal D2 dopamine receptor binding sites (457 $\pm$ 38 fmoles/mg protein) than the older control group (355 $\pm$ 20 fmoles/mg protein). In fact, the old running group had striatal D2 dopamine receptor numbers similar to those of the younger control group (429 $\pm$ 21 fmoles/mg protein). Thus, chronic physical activity appears to exert a protective effect on D2 dopamine receptors during the lifespan (MacRae, Spirduso, Walters, et al., 1987).

In addition, the steady-state levels of dopamine and its metabolites did not differ significantly between the younger control group and the older running group; however, the older control group showed significantly higher levels. It appears that the striatal dopamine measures of the older running group were more similar to those of the younger control group than to those of the older control group. Thus, exercise training may selectively postpone changes in dopamine metabolism over the lifespan. This is of particular importance because the nigrostriatal dopamine system has been shown to deteriorate somewhat selectively with age.

SUGGESTED MECHANISMS

Some evidence supports the idea that regular physical activity can affect the integrity of the CNS in older organisms, both behaviorally and physiologically. Several mechanisms have been suggested to explain these effects. As detailed above, daily bouts of physical activity may allow the nigrostriatal dopamine system to maintain its functional integrity through old age. The effects of physical activity on a variety of neurotransmitter systems should be examined, as well as the interactions among the different neurotransmitter systems in various areas of the aging brain.

A second possible mechanism through which physical activity may affect CNS integrity is its effect on cerebral blood flow and/or cerebral metabolism in the older organism. Though total cerebral blood flow appears to remain constant with physical activity, regional changes in cerebral blood flow and cerebral metabolism have been demonstrated. Mazziotta, Phelps, Carson, and Kuhl (1982) reported a progressive decline in overall cerebral glucose metabolism in young adults when sensory inputs were reduced (vision or audition was reduced artificially). Perhaps the decline in cerebral metabolism in the older brain is due to a decrease in sensory input with age; therefore, physical activity may provide the extra sensory stimulation needed to maintain cerebral metabolism levels similar to those of young adults.

Theories of arousal and attention may be used to explain the physical activity effects on behavioral functioning of the older organism. It has been suggested that the elderly are underaroused and have selective attention deficits (Poon, 1985). Perhaps an increase in arousal, as occurs during exercise, results in a narrowing of attention to those components of a task that are central to rapid and accurate performance. The maintenance of an optimal level of arousal would allow the CNS to function more effectively in a variety of tasks.

Though the effects of aging on CNS function are numerous and well documented, recent evidence suggests that some of these effects are modifiable through lifestyle choices such as regular physical activity. Though the evidence is not plentiful, the older physically active organism does appear to exhibit many of the physiological and behavioral characteristics of a younger organism in terms of CNS function. More evidence is needed to clarify which aspects of the CNS aging are modifiable by physical activity and which aspects are not. Physical activity may be one of the most powerful interventions currently available for combating the deterioration in functional capacity that occurs with the aging of the CNS.

REFERENCES

BHASKARAN, D., & Radha, E. (1983). Monoamine levels and monoamine oxidase activity in different regions of rat brain as a function of age. *Mechanism of Ageing and Development, 23*, 151-160.

BIRREN, J.E., & Schaie, K.W. (1985). *The handbook of the psychology of aging.* New York: Van Nostrand Reinhold.

BIRREN, J.E., Woods, A.M., & Williams, M.V. (1979). Speed of behavior as an indicator of age changes and the integrity of the nervous system. In F. Hoffmeister, C. Muller, & H.P. Krause (Eds.), *Brain function in old age* (pp. 10-44). New York: Springer-Verlag.

BIRREN, J.E., & Zarit, J.M. (1984). Concepts of health, behavior and aging. In J.E. Birren & J. Livingston (Eds.), *Cognition, stress, and aging* (pp. 1-20). Englewood Cliffs, NJ: Prentice Hall.

BROWN, B.S., Payne, T., Chang, K., Moore, G., Krebs, P., & Martin, W. (1979). Chronic response of rat brain norepinephrine and serotonin levels to endurance training. *Journal of Applied Physiology, 46*, 19-23.

BROWN, B.S., & Van Huss, W. (1973). Exercise and rat brain catecholamines. *Journal of Applied Physiology, 34*, 664-669.

BUELL, S.J., & Coleman, P.D. (1979). Dendritic growth in the aged human brain and failure of growth in senile dementia. *Science, 206*, 854-856.

CLARKSON, P. (1978). The effect of age and activity level on simple and choice fractionated response time. *Applied Physiology, 40*, 17-25.

CONNER, J.R., Beban, S.E., Hopper, P.A., Hansen, B., & Diamond, M.C. (1982). A Golgi study of the superficial pyramidal cells in the somatosensory cortex of socially reared old adult rats. *Experimental Neurology, 76*, 35-45.

CONNER, J.R., & Diamond, M.C. (1982). A comparison of dendritic spine number and type on pyramidal neurons of the visual cortex of old adult rats from social or isolated environments. *Journal of Comparative Neurology, 210*, 99-106.

CONNER, J.R., Wang, E.C., & Diamond, M.C. (1982). Increased length of terminal dendritic segments in old adult rats; somatosensory cortex: An environmentally induced response. *Experimental Neurology, 78*, 466-470.

DASTUR, D.K., Lane, M.H., Hansen, D.B., Kety, S.S., Butler, R.N., Perlin, S., & Sokoloff, L. (1963). Effects of aging on cerebral circulation and metabolism in man. In *Human aging: A biological and behavioral study* (PHS publication #986). Washington, DC: U.S. Government Printing Office.

DeCASTRO, J.M., & Duncan, G. (1985). Operantly conditioned running: Effects on brain catecholamine concentrations and receptor densities in the rat. *Pharmacology, Biochemistry, and Behavior, 23*, 495-500.

DUSTMAN, R.E., Ruhling, R.O., Russell, E.M., Shearer, D.E., Bonekat, W., Shigeoka, J.W., Wood, J.S., & Bradford, D.C. (1984). Aerobic exercise training and improved neuropsychological function of older individuals. *Neurobiology of Aging, 5*, 35-42.

FINCH, C.E. (1976). The regulation of physiological changes during mammalian aging. *Quarterly Reviews of Biology, 51*, 49-83.

FINCH, C.E., Randall, P.K., & Marshall, J.F. (1981). Aging and basal gangliar functions. *Annual Reviews of Gerontology and Geriatrics, 2*, 49-87.

FINCH, C.E., & Schneider, E.L. (1985). *The handbook of the biology of aging.* New York: Van Nostrand Reinhold.

FOREMAN, D.L., Snaders, M., & Bloor, C.M. (1976). Total and regional cerebral blood flow during moderate and severe exercise in miniature swine. *Journal of Applied Physiology, 40*, 191-195.

GILLIAM, P.E., Spirduso, W.W., Martin, T.P., Walters, T.J., Wilcox, R.E., & Farrar, R.P. (1984). The effects of exercise training on [3H]-spiperone binding in rat striatum. *Pharmacology, Biochemistry, and Behavior, 20*, 863-867.

GLOBUS, M., Melamed, E., Keren, A., Tzivoni, D., Granot, C., Lavy, S., & Stern, S. (1983). Effect of exercise on cerebral circulation. *Journal of Cerebral Blood Flow and Metabolism*, **3**, 287-290.

GROSS, P.M., Marcus, M.L., & Heistad, D.D. (1980). Regional distribution of cerebral blood flow during exercise in dogs. *Journal of Applied Physiology*, **48**, 213-217.

HERHOLZ, K., Buskies, W., Rist, M., Pawlik, G., Hollmann, W., & Heiss, W.D. (1987). Regional cerebral blood flow in man at rest and during exercise. *Journal of Neurology*, **234**, 9-13.

HUGHES, J.R. (1984). Psychological effects of habitual aerobic exercise: A critical review. *Preventive Medicine*, **13**, 66-78.

KLEINERMAN, J., & Sancetta, S. (1955). Effect of mild steady state exercise on cerebral and general hemodynamics of normal untrained subjects. *Journal of Clinical Investigations*, **34**, 945-946.

MacRAE, P.G., Spirduso, W.W., Cartee, G.D., Farrar, R.P., & Wilcox, R.E. (1987). Endurance training effects on striatal D2 dopamine receptor binding and striatal dopamine metabolite levels. *Neuroscience Letters*, **79**, 138-144.

MacRAE, P.G., Spirduso, W.W., Walters, T.J., Farrar, R.P., & Wilcox, R.E. (1987). Endurance training effects on striatal D2 dopamine receptor binding and striatal dopamine metabolites in presenescent older rats. *Psychopharmacology*, **92**, 236-240.

MAZZIOTTA, J.C., Phelps, M.E., Carson, R.E., & Kuhl, D.E. (1982). Tomographic mapping of human cerebral metabolism: Sensory deprivition. *Annals of Neurology*, **12**, 435-444.

McGEER, P.L., McGeer, E.G., & Suzuki, J.S. (1977). Aging and extrapyramidal function. *Archives of Neurology*, **34**, 33-35.

PANNIER, J.L., & Leusen, I. (1977). Regional blood flow in response to exercise in conscious dogs. *Journal of Applied Physiology*, **36**, 255-265.

PENG, M.T., & Lee, L.R. (1979). Regional differences of neuron loss of rat brain in old age. *Gerontology*, **25**, 305-311.

POON, L.W. (1985). Differences in human memory with aging: Nature, causes, and clinical implications. In J.E. Birren & K.W. Schaie (Eds.), *Handbook of the psychology of aging* (pp. 427-462). New York: Van Nostrand Reinhold.

POWELL, K.E., & Paffenbarger, R.S., Jr. (1985). Workshop on epidemiologic and public health aspects of physical activity and exercise: A summary. *Journal of the United States Public Health Service*, **100**, 118-125.

RIKLI, R., & Busch, S. (1986). Motor performance of women as a function of age and physical activity level. *Journal of Gerontology*, **41**, 645-649.

SALTHOUSE, T.A. (1985). Speed of behavior and its implications for cognition. In J.E. Birren & K.W. Schaie (Eds.), *Handbook of the psychology of aging* (pp. 400-426). New York: Van Nostrand Reinhold.

SAMORAJSKI, T. (1977). Central neurotransmitter substances and aging: A review. *Journal of the American Geriatrics Society*, **25**, 337-348.

SAMORAJSKI, T., Delaney, C., Durham, L., Ordy, J.M., Johnson, J.A., & Dunlap, W.P. (1985). Effect of exercise on longevity, body weight, locomotor performance, and passive-avoidance memory of C57BL/6J mice. *Neurobiology of Aging,* **6**, 17-24.

SCHEIBEL, M.E., Lindsay, R.D., Tomiyasu, U., & Scheibel, A.B. (1975). Progressive dendritic changes in aging human cortex. *Experimental Neurology,* **47**, 392-403.

SCHEIBEL, M.E., Lindsay, R.D., Tomiyasu, U., & Scheibel, A.B. (1976). Progressive dentritic changes in the aging human limbic system. *Experimental Neurology,* **53**, 420-430.

SCHEIBEL, M.E., Tomiyasu, U., & Scheibel, A.B. (1977). The aging human Betz cell. *Experimental Neurology,* **56**, 598-609.

SEVERSON, J.A., & Finch, C.E. (1980). Reduced dopaminergic binding during aging in the rodent striatum. *Brain Research,* **192**, 147-162.

SMITH, C.B. (1984). Aging and changes in cerebral energy metabolism. *Trends in Neuroscience,* **7**, 203-208.

SMITH, C.B., Goochee, C., Rapoport, S.I., & Sokoloff, L. (1980). Effects of aging on local rates of cerebral glucose utilization in rats. *Brain,* **103**, 351-365.

SPIRDUSO, W.W. (1975). Reaction and movement time as a function of age and physical activity level. *Journal of Gerontology,* **30**, 435-440.

SPIRDUSO, W.W. (1980). Physical fitness, aging, and psychomotor speed: A review. *Journal of Gerontology,* **35**, 850-865.

SPIRDUSO, W.W. (1983). Exercise and the aging brain. *Research Quarterly for Exercise and Sport,* **54**, 208-218.

SPIRDUSO, W.W. (1984). Exercise as a factor in aging motor behavior plasticity. In M.L. Pollock, J.H. Wilmore, & S.M. Fox (Eds.), *Exercise in health and disease* (pp. 89-99). Philadelphia: W.B. Saunders.

SPIRDUSO, W.W., & Clifford, P. (1978). Replication of age and physical activity effects on reaction and movement time. *Journal of Gerontology,* **33**, 26-30.

SPIRDUSO, W.W., MacRae, H.H., MacRae, P.G., Prewitt, J., & Osborne, L. (1988). Exercise effects on aged motor function. *Annals of the New York Academy of Sciences,* **515**, 363-375.

TOMPOROWSKI, P.D., & Ellis, N.R. (1986). Effects of exercise on cognitive processes: A review. *Psychological Bulletin,* **99**, 338-346.

VIJAYASHANKER, N., & Brody, H. (1979). A quantitative study of the pigmented neurons in the nuclei locus coeruleus and subcoeruleus in man as related to aging. *Journal of Neuropathology and Experimental Neurology,* **38**, 490-497.

WANG, H.S., & Busse, E.W. (1969). EEG of healthy old persons—A longitudinal study. I. Dominant background activity and occipital rhythm. *Journal of Gerontology,* **24**, 419-426.

WANG, H.S., Obrist, W.D., & Busse, E.W. (1970). Neurophysiological correlates of the intellectual function of elderly persons living in the community. *American Journal of Psychiatry,* **126**, 1205-1212.

ZOBL, E.G., Talmers, F.N., Christensen, R.C., & Baer, L.J. (1965). Effect of exercise on the cerebral circulation and metabolism. *Journal of Applied Physiology,* **20**, 1289-1293.

Variation in Fat Distribution With Age and Health Implications

Claude Bouchard and Jean-Pierre Després
Laval University

It has long been recognized that excess body fat or obesity is a risk factor for cardiovascular disease. Excess body fat is accompanied by an increased susceptibility to a variety of clinical disorders and a high mortality rate (Andres, 1985; Osler, 1987; Simopoulos & Van Itallie, 1984). In some studies, however, the link between excessive body weight and morbidity or mortality was rather weak, and it raised some doubt about the obese state as a true risk factor independent from other risk factors. It appears that two main reasons could explain this uncertainty in the data.

First, it was shown that the duration of the obese state, that is, the number of years during which an excessive body weight is maintained, was an important variable. Data from the Framingham study (Feinleib, 1985) and the Manitoba study of Canadian Air Force pilots (Rabkin, Mathewson, & Hsu, 1977) indicated that the detrimental effects of obesity became more apparent when the obese state had been maintained for about 10 years or more. Thus, the notion that a relatively long incubation period is necessary for the complications of obesity to become manifest is an important one. From several large-scale life insurance and prospective studies, it is believed that the relative risk of death reaches about 1.5 when long-term obese individuals are compared to lean subjects. In general, obesity is associated with a higher death rate from coronary heart disease, cerebrovascular disease, type II diabetes mellitus, hypertensive diseases, and endometrial cancer as well as postmenopausal breast cancer and their related complications.

Second, it is increasingly recognized that one must consider not only the amount of excess fat in assessing the risk associated with obesity but also the topography of adipose tissue per se. Vague (1956) was the first to recognize that the male pattern of fat distribution in obesity was characterized by a higher propensity to metabolic complications. Abdominal obesity (often referred to as android obesity) is progressively being recognized as a type of obesity that carries a greater risk than excess body fat by itself. Three recent symposia held in Marseilles, London, and Québec have dealt with the topic of body fat distribution and its health correlates (Bouchard & Johnston, 1988; Norgan, 1985; Vague, Björntorp, Guy-Grand, Rebuffé-Scrive, & Vague, 1985). The clinical and epidemiological evidence reviewed at these symposia, particularly from five prospective studies,

78

has made clear that abdominal obesity is characterized by a relative risk of about 2.0 for morbid conditions and mortality compared to lean controls. This relative risk is comparable in magnitude to that entailed by smoking, hypertension, and hypercholesterolemia for cardiovascular disease. The five prospective studies that have included an assessment of fat distribution are identified in Table 1.

Our task in the context of the present symposium on aging is to discuss the changes taking place in fat distribution with age, with a focus on abdominal fat, and the relevant alterations in the metabolic profile. This is an important topic to consider in the study of the biology of aging and the impact of regular physical activity. It is well known that the prevalence of obesity increases with age in both genders. For instance, in the Canadian population less than 3% of the females in the 20- to 29-year age group have a body mass index (BMI) of 30 and above, whereas about 15% reach that level of obesity in the 50- to 70-years-of-age category (Fitness and Amateur Sport Canada, 1986). Not only does the population exhibit a higher prevalence of obese individuals up to about 70 years of age, after which there are fewer of them, but the prevalence of abdominal obesity is also increasing as revealed by skinfold and circumference data from the same Canadian epidemiological study. In other words, in each gender three important and correlated risk factors are operating concomitantly, namely age, excess body weight, and abdominal fat.

Table 1

Prospective Studies That Have Reported
Associations Between Body Fat Distribution and Cardiovascular Disease

Study	Sample size	Age range	Body fat distribution variable	Years of follow-up
Gothenburg	1462 F	38-60	WHR[1]	12
Gothenburg	792 M	54	WHR	13
Framingham	2420 F	36-68	Subscapular skinfold	22
	1834 M	36-38		
Paris Prospective Study	7746 M	52-53	Trunk fat component[2]	6.6
Honolulu Heart Program	7692 M	—	Subscapular skinfold	12

[1]Waist-to-hip circumferences ratio.
[2]Derived from principal component analysis.

In this review, after discussing the methods to assess fat topography, we will describe the changes in body fat distribution with age. These sections will be followed by a review of the metabolic alterations related to abdominal obesity in the context of aging, along with the potential mechanisms involved. Finally, the contribution of genetic factors, nutrition, and exercise in regional fat distribution will be discussed.

ASSESSMENT OF REGIONAL BODY FAT DISTRIBUTION

In the context of this paper, it would seem useful to distinguish between the following three concepts pertaining to the assessment of fat topography in humans (Bouchard, 1988c). *Total body fat* is defined as the absolute amount of fat (mostly adipose tissue) in the body. Its relative contribution to total body mass, that is, percent of the body as fat, is also often considered. The fat mass of the body can be assessed using a variety of direct procedures including underwater weighing to measure body density, which is then converted to percent fat and fat mass, K^{40} content of the body to estimate the proportion of lean tissue and then the fat component, total body electrical conductivity (TOBEC), various isotope dilution methods, and some others.

Fat distribution represents the amount of fat in various compartments or regions of the body. It can be described in absolute or in relative terms. *Fat patterning* is the notion used when describing the relative anatomical location of subcutaneous fat. It is usually expressed in terms of the principal components or the factors extracted from a correlation matrix of skinfold measurements by principal component or factorial analyses.

The main concept of interest here is fat distribution as opposed to total body fat and subcutaneous fat patterning. In the literature, body fat distribution is presented as (a) upper body versus lower body fat, (b) trunk versus extremity fat, (c) trunk versus lower extremity fat, (d) upper trunk versus lower trunk fat, (e) upper extremity versus lower extremity fat, (f) subcutaneous fat versus total fat mass, (g) subcutaneous fat versus visceral fat, and (h) subcutaneous abdominal fat versus visceral abdominal fat. Each of these characteristics has been described in relative or absolute size depending on the views of the authors (Bouchard, 1988c). A growing body of clinical evidence indicates that the emphasis should be put on the trunk, particularly lower trunk or abdominal fat, when considering the metabolic and health implications of individual differences and of variation over time in fat distribution.

Skinfolds, circumferences, ultrasound pictures, radiographs, and computed axial tomography (CT scan) have been used in various ways to assess fat distribution. In the case of skinfolds, ratios of selected measurements have been primarily used. We have made extensive use of a trunk (sum of 3 skinfolds) to extremity (sum of 3 skinfolds) skinfold ratio, and of a subcutaneous fat (sum of 6 skinfolds) to total fat mass (from underwater weighing) ratio in epidemiological (Després, Allard, Tremblay, Talbot, & Bouchard, 1985; Després, Tremblay, Pérusse, Leblanc, & Bouchard, 1988; Després, Tremblay, Theriault, et al., in press), genetic (Bouchard, 1988b; Bouchard, Savard, Després, Tremblay, & Leblanc, 1985), and exercise-training studies (Després, Bouchard, Tremblay, Savard, & Marcotte, 1985; Després, Moorjani, Tremblay, et al., 1988).

Earlier, Vague (1947, 1956) had used skinfolds and circumferences in the brachial and the femoral regions to compute the brachio-femoral adipomuscular ratio, one of the first indices of fat distribution. The same issue was approached in a simplified way by Kissebah and his colleagues who, building further upon the early research of Vague, proposed to use the ratio of the waist circumference (W) to the hip circumference (H), the so-called WHR (Kissebah et al., 1982; Kissebah, Peiris, & Evans, 1988). Along these lines, Ashwell, Cole, and Dixon

(1985) had proposed to use a waist-to-thigh circumference ratio. Ultrasound imaging has the potential to distinguish the superficial and the deep component of adipose tissue in a given body area, but it has not been used to any extent for this purpose. It has rather been used to assess the amount of fat in a given body segment (Booth, Godddard, & Paton, 1966).

Radiographs can also be used to assess fat distribution (Borkan & Norris, 1977), but more recently the emphasis has shifted to CT scan data. Computed tomography has proven to be a reliable method to assess fat distribution over the body and to distinguish the subcutaneous from the deep fat depot in various parts of the body (Borkan et al., 1982; Borkan, Hults, Gerzof, Robbins, & Silbert, 1983; Enzi et al., 1986; Ferland et al., 1988; Grauer, Moss, Cann, & Goldberg, 1984; Kvist, Sjöström, & Tylen, 1986; Seidell et al., 1987; Sjöström, 1988; Sjöström, Kvist, Cederblad, & Tylen, 1986; Sjöström, Kvist, & Tylen, 1985; Tokunaga, Matsuzawa, Ishikawa, & Tarui, 1983). The studies pioneered by Sjöström and his colleagues indicate that visceral adipose tissue represents about 8% of the total CT scan adipose tissue in women, but more than 20% in men. If the amount of visceral adipose tissue in the abdominal cavity is the critical variable for all practical purposes, it is significantly correlated with abdominal skinfold ($r \approx 0.6$), waist circumference ($r \approx 0.8$), and WHR ($r \approx 0.6$ to 0.8) in both sexes (Ferland et al., 1988; Sjöström, 1988). Some of these relationships are summarized in Table 2.

It should be noted that the commonly used WHR was the anthropometric variable that displayed the highest association with the proportion of visceral fat in a sample of 51 obese women that we recently studied (Ferland et al., 1988). As visceral fat appears to be important in the association between body fat distribution and health, this relation of intra-abdominal fat to WHR might help explain the association frequently reported between WHR and cardiovascular disease.

Table 2

Fat Distribution From CT Scan and Anthropometry in 51 Premenopausal Obese Women (from the data of Ferland et al.)

	Amount of visceral fat[a]	Proportion of visceral fat[b]
Fat mass (kg)[c]	.72	.17
Sum 7 skinfolds	.62	.28*
Abdominal skinfold	.65	.38**
Waist circumference	.76	.26
WHR	.55	.49***

[a]From the CT scan at L4/L5 level. [b]Ratio of visceral to total adipose tissue at L4/L5 level. [c]From underwater weighing.
*$p<0.05$; **$p<0.01$; ***$p<0.001$.

VARIATION IN FAT DISTRIBUTION WITH AGE

In the context of this symposium, one would like to know whether there are changes in fat distribution with age. First, one should recognize that individual differences in fat distribution characteristics are considerable, such that group data may at times be misleading. Second, we have found a significant genetic effect in various indicators of fat distribution amounting to about 25% of the phenotypic variance (Bouchard, 1985, 1987, 1988b; Bouchard, Pérusse, et al., 1988). This result implies that some individuals are more likely than others to store fat in a given region or compartment of the body than in other areas. Thus, a given individual may behave quite differently from a sample of subjects in terms of site of preferential fat deposition because of inherited characteristics.

The study of fat distribution during growth reveals some interesting trends (Malina & Bouchard, 1988). Fat mass increases at a faster rate than subcutaneous fat during childhood. This trend continues through adolescence in girls only. Boys accumulate relatively more fat on the trunk during adolescence, which is accentuated by a reduction in subcutaneous fat on the extremities. In girls, subcutaneous fat on both the trunk and extremities increases at a similar pace during adolescence. Early and late maturing girls do not differ in subcutaneous fat distribution whereas early maturing boys have relatively more subcutaneous fat on the trunk than late maturing boys (Malina & Bouchard, 1988).

As shown by Sjöström (1988), the amount of visceral fat varies considerably in adults, with a mean value of about 8% of total CT adipose volume in women (range 4–14%) and 20% in men (range 9–34%). The early studies based on skinfolds and radiographs had suggested that internal fat was increasing with age while subcutaneous fat was either declining or unchanged (Borkan & Norris, 1977). More recent studies using CT scan to assess abdominal fat and its visceral component have provided more direct evidence for this trend. Thus Borkan et al. (1983) have shown that visceral fat surface obtained from one abdominal scan increased significantly with age, representing 38% of the abdominal fat area in 46-year-old males but 47% in 69-year-old males (Table 3). This was found despite the fact that subcutaneous fat measurements from various sites were lower in the older subjects than in young men.

Enzi et al. (1986), also using CT scan methodology, found that visceral fat area (upper kidney level) increased with age from 20 to 60 years and above in both genders. Their data also indicate that subjects with a higher BMI also have a larger visceral fat component (Table 4). These alterations in abdominal visceral fat area were not related to the changes in the CT abdominal subcutaneous fat area, as the latter was higher in females and in the overweight subjects but was not affected by age.

In summary, these data indicate that abdominal fat increases with age in both sexes but more so in men than in women. On the average, men have more visceral fat in the abdominal compartment than women and they reach even higher values with age. Overweight and obese individuals of both sexes have more abdominal visceral fat at all ages.

METABOLIC CHANGES ASSOCIATED
WITH BODY FAT DISTRIBUTION

To our knowledge, no study has considered simultaneously the changes with aging in regional fat distribution and the changes in the metabolic and risk profiles.

Table 3

Comparison of Younger (*N* = 21) and Older (*N* = 20) Men for Body Composition and Fat Distribution[a]

Variable	Young M	Young SD	Old M	Old SD	T test
Age	46	3	69	4	
Body weight (kg)	82	10	74	8	2.9**
Percent fat	30	7	32	6	0.7
CT umbilicus fat (cm²)					
Subcutaneous	206	96	172	40	1.5
Visceral	126	50	158	57	2.0*
% Visceral	38	9	47	13	2.4*
CT upper leg fat (cm²)	229	27	185	25	5.4**
CT upper arm fat (cm²)	86	13	80	10	1.7

[a]*Note.* Adapted from Borkan et al., 1983.
*$p < 0.05$; **$p < 0.01$.

Table 4

CT Visceral Fat Area (CM²) in the Abdomen (Upper Kidney Level) With Age, Gender, and Body Mass Index

	Age groups (years) 20–30	40–59	>60
Normal weight subjects (BMI≤26)			
Males	56	74	94
Females	37	39	57
Overweight subjects (BMI>26)			
Males	113	185	180
Females	82	94	124

Note. Adapted from Enzi et al., 1986.

We therefore have to assume that the relationships between the major features of fat distribution and the metabolic characteristics of interest are essentially the same in the young or middle-aged adults and the older individuals. We also have to assume that the experimentally induced changes in fat distribution in younger individuals can help us to understand the age-related alterations observed when one gets older.

Although numerous recent studies have reported significant associations between body fat distribution and coronary heart disease and related mortality, the mechanisms responsible for this relationship remain to be established. However, numerous reports have shown that the topography of adipose tissue was associated with risk factors for cardiovascular disease such as diabetes, changes in plasma lipid and lipoprotein levels, and hypertension (Anderson et al., 1988; Blair, Habicht, Sims, Sylwester, & Abraham, 1984; Després, Allard, et al., 1985; Després, Tremblay, & Bouchard, 1988; Després, Tremblay, Pérusse, et al., 1988; Després, Tremblay, Thériault, et al., in press; Hartz, Rupley, Kalkhoff, & Rimm, 1983; Kalkhoff, Hartz, Rupley, Kissebah, & Kelber, 1983; Kissebah et al., 1982; Krotkiewski, Björntorp, Sjöström, & Smith, 1983; Vague, 1956).

Body Fat Distribution, Hyperinsulinemia, Insulin Resistance, and Diabetes

As early as 1956, Vague reported that individuals with an android distribution of body fat were more metabolically affected than obese individuals with a gynoid distribution of body fat. More recently, Kissebah et al. (1982) reported a greater incidence of hyperinsulinemia and glucose intolerance in upper-body obese women compared to lower-body obese women. In a comprehensive survey of 15,532 obese women, Hartz et al. (1983) showed that obese subjects with excessive upper body fat had a relative risk of diabetes more than 10 times that of normal women with peripheral fat accumulation. These results are in concordance with other studies reporting that body fat topography was associated with plasma insulin and glucose responses to a glucose challenge (Evans, Hoffman, Kalkhoff, & Kissebah, 1984; Kalkhoff et al., 1983; Krotkiewski et al., 1983). In addition, a recent longitudinal study has clearly indicated that the localization of body fat could predict, over a 13-year period, the development of diabetes (Ohlson et al., 1985). These results suggest that body fat distribution is as important as obesity in terms of its effect on glucose and insulin metabolism, and that the link between body fat topography and diabetes could be considered one of the mechanisms by which body fat topography is associated with cardiovascular disease.

Sparrow, Borkan, Gerzof, Wisniewski, and Silbert (1986) showed that intra-abdominal fat was a significant correlate of plasma glucose levels 2 hours after glucose ingestion. As the proportion of visceral fat increases with age (Borkan et al., 1983), whether glucose intolerance associated with intra-abdominal fat accumulation is an age-related or age-independent phenomenon remains to be established. Fujioka, Matsuzawa, Tokunaga, and Tarui (1987) have reported that glucose tolerance was positively correlated with the proportion of visceral fat, and that this relationship was independent from the body mass index and from age. Although this study included men and women with a wide age range, these results suggest that intra-abdominal fat is indeed associated with glucose intolerance and that this effect is independent from the increase in visceral fat observed with age. In a sample of obese women homogeneous in terms of age, we have also observed that intra-abdominal fat accumulation was the critical variable in the association between body fat distribution and glucose tolerance (Després, Nadeau, et al., 1988). Therefore, due to its deleterious effect on carbohydrate metabolism, intra-abdominal fat accumulation should be considered as a health hazard.

The mechanism by which body fat distribution affects glucose metabolism is not fully understood, but the possibilities are described in Figure 1. Björntorp

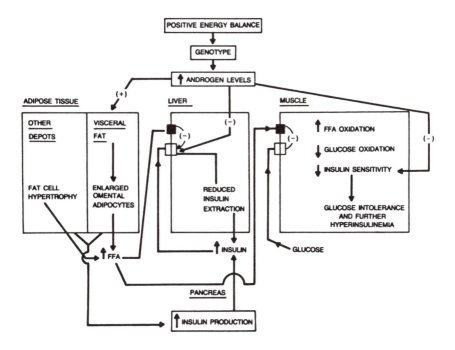

Figure 1 — Potential mechanisms accounting for the relation of abdominal obesity to aberrations in glucose tolerance and plasma insulin levels. Enlarged abdominal adipose cells, especially omental adipocytes, which are hyperlipolytic and resistant to the antilipolytic action of insulin, liberate higher concentrations of free fatty acids into the portal circulation impairing hepatic insulin extraction and reducing peripheral glucose uptake. Such a condition may contribute to the establishment of glucose intolerance and hyperinsulinemia, potentially leading to type II diabetes mellitus if environmental and genetic factors are present. Adapted from Kissebah et al. (1985, 1988) and from Després, Moorjani, Ferland, et al. (1988).

(1984, 1985) and Kissebah, Evans, Peiris, and Wilson (1985) have suggested that enlarged intra-abdominal adipocytes, which have a very lively lipolysis, release high quantities of free fatty acids (FFA) into the portal circulation, exposing the liver and peripheral tissues to high FFA concentrations that impair glucose uptake. Increased portal FFA concentration could reduce insulin clearance by the liver, producing peripheral hyperinsulinemia that could lead to insulin resistance. Indeed, Peiris, Mueller, Smith, Struve, and Kissebah (1986) have shown that abdominal obesity was associated with a reduced hepatic extraction of insulin.

Another possibility is that high levels of visceral fat accumulation and insulin resistance are due to hormonal changes (increase in androgen levels) affecting both the body fat distribution and carbohydrate metabolism. From the available literature (Evans et al., 1984; Kissebah et al., 1985), it appears reasonable to propose that both mechanisms are involved in the impairment of glucose metabolism associated with body fat distribution.

Body Fat Distribution
and Plasma Lipoprotein-Lipid Levels

Disturbances in carbohydrate homeostasis and increased susceptibility to diabetes, however, are not the only factors responsible for the association between body fat distribution and cardiovascular disease. Indeed, since the early study of Albrink and Meigs (1965) that reported a positive association between fat located in the trunk and plasma triglyceride levels, many reports have indicated that body fat distribution was associated with plasma lipid and lipoprotein levels. Using the waist-to-hip ratio (WHR) as an anthropometric estimate of the proportion of abdominal fat, Kissebah et al. (1982), Krotkiewski et al. (1983), and Evans et al. (1984) have also shown that abdominal obesity was related to high plasma triglyceride levels. We have also reported, as shown in Table 5, that a high proportion of abdominal fat was associated not only with high serum triglyceride levels but also with low serum HDL-cholesterol levels (Després, Allard, et al., 1985).

Further analyses indicated that this relationship between abdominal fat and serum HDL-cholesterol was partly independent from serum triglyceride levels and unexplained by variations in total adiposity (Després, Tremblay, Pérusse, Leblanc, & Bouchard, 1988). Indeed, Table 6 presents analysis of variance results showing that, in a sample of 429 men, the variance in serum triglyceride and HDL-cholesterol levels is solely explained by the amount of abdominal fat and not by total fatness.

Table 7 indicates that after correction for total fatness there was a significant partial correlation between the amount of abdominal fat and serum HDL-cholesterol levels, whereas after control for abdominal fat there was no significant association between total fatness and serum HDL-cholesterol levels, emphasizing the important effect of abdominal obesity per se on lipoprotein metabolism.

Many recent studies have confirmed this finding of a negative association

Table 5

Correlations Between Body Fat Mass, Various Skinfold Measurements, and Serum Lipid and HDL-Cholesterol Levels in Men ($N = 238$)

Variable	CHOL	TG	HDL-CHOL	HDL-CHOL/CHOL
Body fat mass	0.21**	0.33**	−0.24**	−0.35**
Sum of 6 skinfolds	0.17*	0.30**	−0.28**	−0.35**
Triceps	0.11	0.19**	−0.21**	−0.26**
Biceps	0.13	0.25**	−0.24**	−0.29**
Subscapular	0.20**	0.33**	−0.32**	−0.40**
Suprailiac	0.07	0.12	−0.15*	−0.18**
Abdomen	0.22**	0.36**	−0.27**	−0.38**
Calf	0.04	0.15*	−0.19**	−0.18**

Note. Adapted from Després et al., 1985.
*$p<0.05$; **$p<0.01$.

Table 6

Analysis of Variance for the Effects of Abdominal Fat and the Body Mass Index on Serum Triglyceride and HDL-Cholesterol Levels in Men (N = 429)

| | | BMI tertiles | | | |
		I	II	III	
Triglycerides					
Abdominal	I	93.8	151.1	134.1	$F = 1.9$
Skinfold	II	157.1	135.7	138.5	n.s.
Tertiles	III	152.9	168.3	186.8	
			$F = 4.8, p < 0.01$		
HDL-CHOL					
Abdominal	I	50.4	46.5	47.4	$F = 2.3$
Skinfold	II	50.5	48.6	48.4	n.s.
Tertiles	III	47.9	42.4	42.4	
			$F = 3.5, p < 0.05$		

Note. Values are in mg/dl; n.s. = not significant. Adapted from Després et al., 1988.

Table 7

Partial Correlation Coefficients for the Independent Associations Between Abdominal Fat, Body Mass Index, and Serum Lipids and Lipoproteins in Men (N = 429)

Variable	Abdominal skinfold (corrected for BMI)	BMI (corrected for abdominal skinfold)
TG	0.17**	0.12**
CHOL	0.09 n.s.	0.12*
HDL-CHOL	−0.12*	−0.07 n.s.
HDL-CHOL/CHOL	−0.16**	−0.14*

Note. Adapted from Després et al., 1988.
*$p < 0.05$; **$p < 0.01$; n.s. = not significant.

between body fat distribution and HDL-cholesterol levels (Anderson et al., 1988; Foster et al., 1987; Haffner, Stern, Hazuda, Pugh, & Patterson, 1987; Kissebah et al., 1985; Terry, Stefanick, Krauss, Haskell, & Wood, 1985). Although body fat distribution appears to be associated with plasma lipoprotein levels, the role of visceral abdominal fat has not been extensively studied. However, we have recently observed that, in a sample of obese women, visceral abdominal fat was negatively correlated with plasma HDL-cholesterol levels (Després, Moorjani, Ferland, et al., 1988), and that this association was independent from age and total adiposity. As low HDL-cholesterol levels are considered a risk factor for coronary heart disease (Castelli, 1984), these results further emphasize the important role of intra-abdominal fat in determining the cardiovascular disease risk. The hypothetical mechanisms for this association have recently been reviewed (Després, Tremblay, & Bouchard, 1988) and are presented in Figure 2.

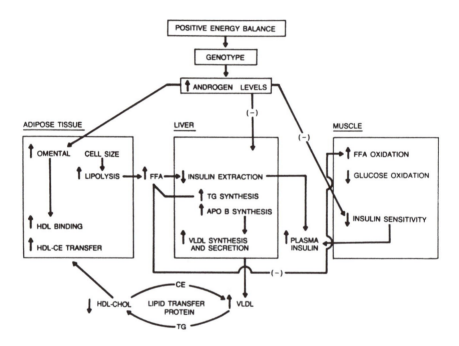

Figure 2 — Potential mechanisms accounting for the association between abdominal obesity and plasma lipoprotein levels. Hyperinsulinemia and high plasma free fatty acid levels produce an increase in hepatic very-low-density lipoprotein (VLDL) secretion. High plasma VLDL levels may cause changes in plasma lipoprotein-lipid composition. In addition, the binding of high density lipoproteins (HDL) to large abdominal fat cells and the preferential cholesterol ester transfer to abdominal adipocytes could reduce the cholesterol content of HDL. The role of adipose tissue and muscle lipoprotein lipase (LPL) in the association between body fat distribution and plasma lipoproteins is not known. As high hepatic lipase (HL) activity is noted in subjects with high unbound androgen levels, HL activity is also probably high in abdominal obesity. The association between body fat distribution and lecithin cholesterol acyl transferase activity is also not known. In addition, the potential association between body fat distribution and liver Apo B, E receptor activity has never been studied. Finally, whether the disproportionate uptake of HDL-cholesterol ester by the abdominal fat cells is unidirectional or represents an exchange process is not known. Adapted from Després et al. (1988).

Body Fat Distribution and Blood Pressure

It also appears that high blood pressure is another factor that should receive attention, as numerous reports have indicated that body fat localization is associated with hypertension (Blair et al., 1984; Després, Tremblay, Thériault, et al., in press; Kalkhoff et al., 1983; Weinsier et al., 1985). Blair et al. (1984) showed that trunk fat had more detrimental effects on blood pressure than peripheral fat. Kalkhoff et al. (1983) reported significant associations between the WHR and blood pressure. Krotkiewski et al. (1983) as well as Weinsier et al. (1985) studied the respective contributions of total body fat and body fat distribution to variations in blood pressure, and both studies reported a significant effect of body fat localization on blood pressure. As blood pressure also increases with age, we controlled for the effects of environmental covariables known to affect blood pressure (including age) and have observed a significant effect of the proportion of trunk fat on the diastolic blood pressure of men (Després, Tremblay, Thériault, et al., in press). Table 8 presents analyses of variance for the effects of total fatness and subcutaneous body fat distribution in a sample of 238 men. Results indicate that a significant portion of the variance in diastolic blood pressure is associated with variation in body fat distribution.

Although all these studies showed an effect of body fat distribution on blood pressure, the mechanism by which these variables are linked will require further study. However, a role for insulin, whose levels are associated with body fat topography, has been proposed (Christlieb, Krolewski, Warram, & Soeldner, 1985; DeFronzo, 1981; Krotkiewski et al., 1979; Landsberg, 1986; Sims & Berchtold, 1982). A preliminary model linking body fat distribution, plasma insulin levels, and blood pressure is illustrated in Figure 3. It is important to men-

Table 8

Analysis of Variance for the Effects of Body Fat Distribution and of Percent Body Fat on Blood Pressure in Men ($N = 238$)

	Lean	Fat	
Diastolic BP			
T/E ratio			
Low	70.3 ± 9.3	76.4 ± 10.9	$F = 14.4$
High	75.3 ± 8.6	78.7 ± 9.3	$p < 0.01$
	$F = 8.4, P < 0.01$		
Systolic BP			
T/E ratio			
Low	115.6 ± 12.0	120.0 ± 13.5	$F = 8.9$
High	116.5 ± 10.4	121.8 ± 13.2	$p < 0.01$
	$F = 0.7$, n.s.		

Note. Values are in mm HG ± SD; n.s. = not significant. Adapted from Després, Tremblay, Thériault, et al., in press.

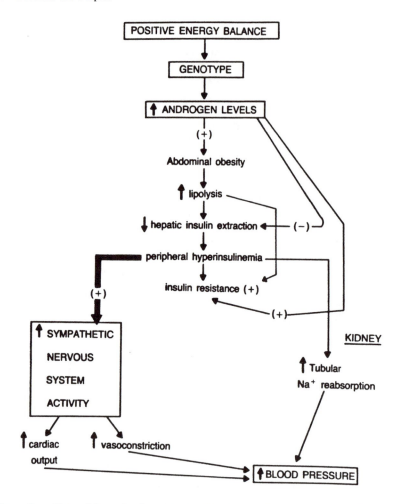

Figure 3 — Potential mechanisms involved in the association between body fat distribution and blood pressure. Adapted from results of Christlieb et al., 1985; DeFronzo, 1981; Kalkhoff et al., 1983; Kissebah et al., 1982, 1985; Krotkiewski et al., 1979, 1983; Landsberg, 1986; Sims & Berchtold, 1982.

tion that blood pressure has been associated with anthropometric measures of body fat distribution only, and its relationship with computed axial tomography measurements of visceral fat will have to be studied.

Body Fat Distribution and Metabolism: A Summary

From the above discussion, it is clear that the strong independent effect of body fat distribution on cardiovascular disease can be explained by the metabolic disturbances observed in abdominal obesity. In addition to the independent effects of insulin resistance and diabetes, of plasma lipoprotein-lipid levels and of hypertension on cardiovascular disease, it should be emphasized that these metabolic complications will probably tend to be further exacerbated in abdominal obesity, and perhaps more so in the aging person. Therefore, the interaction of these risk factors should markedly increase the probability of a cardiovascular accident in these individuals. Finally, results from computed axial tomography indicate that visceral abdominal fat accumulation is a critical variable to consider in the delineation of the mechanisms linking body fat distribution to metabolic complications.

GENETICS AND FAT DISTRIBUTION

Beyond the events of sexual maturation, once the adult fat distribution characteristics have been attained, the absolute amount of fat in the various body compartments is thought to be modulated primarily according to the long-term conditions of the individual's energy balance. Under persistent positive energy balance, fat deposition will result, while fat mobilization will be the consequence of long-term negative energy balance. Assuming that the individuals in the population are more or less in energy balance, can one detect a genetic effect accounting for some of the variations seen in fat distribution?

We will attempt to answer this question for several indicators of fat distribution. Skinfold and underwater weighing measurements were obtained in a maximum of 1,698 individuals from 409 families from the Québec city area (Bouchard, 1985, 1988a; Bouchard, Pérusse, Leblanc, Tremblay, & Thériault, in press). The following indicators of fat distribution were considered: (a) the sum of the abdominal plus the suprailiac skinfolds, (b) the ratio of the sum of the abdominal plus the suprailiac skinfolds divided by the sum of the triceps and the medial calf skinfolds, and (c) the sum of six skinfolds (biceps, subscapular, triceps, medial calf, suprailiac, and abdominal) divided by fat mass in kg. These three indicators of fat distribution were available in pairs of spouses (N=maximum of 348 pairs), foster parent–adopted child (N=322), siblings by adoption (N=120), first-degree cousins (N=95), uncle/aunt–nephew/niece (N=88), parent–natural child (N=1,239), siblings by descent (N=370), dizygotic twins (N=69), and monozygotic twins (N=87).

Data were analyzed under two conditions: after adjustment by a regression procedure for the effects of age and gender, and after adjustment for age, gender, and total amount of subcutaneous fat using the sum of six skinfolds for that purpose. The first strategy allows us to estimate the genetic effect in fat distribution regardless of total fat, while the second strategy provides an estimate of the genetic effect in fat distribution after control over the level of subcutaneous fatness.

Genetic epidemiologists have developed several methods for estimating the additive genetic effect from data gathered on several kinds of biological relatives and relatives by adoption. One approach is to use a path analysis procedure specially designed to estimate the biological inheritance component and other relevant parameters for quantitative traits such as body fat distribution. We have applied one of these methods, the BETA path analysis model (Cloninger, Rice, & Reich, 1979), to data that were gathered in our laboratory on the nine kinds of relatives identified above. Some of the results are summarized in Table 9. The additive genetic effect is quite small for the amount of fat in the abdominal area (h^2 = .10), but it increases to 0.25 when data are adjusted for the total amount of subcutaneous fat. In other words, the genetic effect is higher and quite significant (25%) when one controls for human variation in level of fatness. These results

Table 9

Total Transmissible Variance Across Generations and its Additive Genetic Component for the Three Indicators of Fat Distribution Without and With Adjustment for Level of Fatness

Variance	Transmissible variance (t^2)	Biological inheritance (h^2)	Cultural inheritance (b^2)	Nontransmissible variance (e^2)	χ^2 (p)
Scores adjusted for age and gender					
Abdominal + suprailiac[a]	.36	.10	.26	.64	15.7 ($p<.01$)
AS/TC ratio	.59	.23	.35	.41	5.2 ($p<.10$)
Sum skinfolds/fat mass	.37	.25	.10	.63	3.0 ($p<.50$)
Scores adjusted for age, gender, and fatness					
Abdominal + suprailiac	.58	.25	.32	.42	2.6 ($p<.50$)
AS/TC ratio	.67	.19	.46	.33	1.5 ($p<.50$)

Note. The BETA path analysis procedure was used to obtain these estimates. Only the full model solution is presented. The fit is acceptable for all variables except[a]. AS/TC ratio obtained from the sum of abdominal and suprailiac skinfolds divided by the sum of triceps and medial calf skinfolds. Adapted from Bouchard, 1988.

indicate that some individuals of either sex undoubtedly have more fat in the lower trunk area as a consequence of undetermined genetic characteristics. On the other hand, the additive genetic effect is also moderately high for the two ratios of fat distribution and remains so with data adjusted for level of fatness, that is, from about 20 to 25%. Taken as a whole, these results indicate that there are genetically determined differences in the regions of the body where fat is preferentially stored, and this effect is seen whether total fatness is taken into consideration or not (Bouchard, 1988).

Let us now turn our attention to a special genetic effect, one that is often known as the genotype (G) and environment (E) interaction effect, or G×E. The G×E effect results from the fact that all individuals (or genotypes) do not respond similarly to changes in E. In the present report, we ask whether such a G×E component exists for body fat distribution when energy balance is systematically manipulated. In other words, are there innate differences in the sensitivity to a positive or a negative energy balance? We believe that there are, as suggested by the study briefly reviewed below.

In our laboratory, Poehlman et al. (1986) subjected six pairs of male MZ twins (i.e., only a maximum of six genotypes were tested) to a 4.2 MJ/day overfeeding stress for 22 consecutive days. Data indicate that adaptation to caloric affluence in terms of fat deposition differed between genotypes but was significantly similar in members of the same MZ pair. Subjects gained weight and fat with overfeeding, but there were considerable interindividual differences in the changes observed. However, these changes were not randomly distributed, as indicated by the presence of significant genotype-overfeeding interactions. Intrapair resemblance in the response to overfeeding was consistently high, as revealed by intraclass coefficients. For instance, a 0.90 intraclass correlation for changes in percent fat was found, indicating that about 90% of the variance in the response was between genotypes, while only about 10% of the variance was within pairs (results not shown). These data suggest that fat deposition in response to caloric affluence is significantly determined by the genotype.

Is there a G×E component for fat distribution when energy balance is systematically manipulated? This question was also considered in our study of six pairs of male MZ twins. Subjects gained weight and fat with overfeeding, but there were considerable interindividual differences in terms of the regional fat deposition (Table 10). For instance, the 0.74 intraclass correlation for changes in the ratio of subcutaneous fat to total fat mass implies that about three quarters of the variance in response were between genotypes, while only 25% of the variance could be found within pairs. These data suggest that not only the amount of fat deposition but also the location of fat deposition in response to caloric affluence are partly determined by the genotype. In other words, there is a G×E effect when exposed to a positive energy balance and some individuals are more at risk than others to deposit fat and to store it in regions that may cause metabolic aberrations.

NONGENETIC FACTORS AND BODY FAT DISTRIBUTION

Nutrition

Although it has been shown that genetic factors are important in body fat distribution, it is rather obvious that environmental factors play a role in the regula-

Table 10

Analysis of Variance and Intraclass Correlation for Fat Distribution Changes Following Short-Term Overfeeding[a]

Variable	Effect of overfeeding (F ratio)[b]	Genotype-overfeeding interaction (F ratio)	Intrapair resemblance in response
Abdominal skinfold	43.5**	3.8	0.58
Suprailiac skinfold	13.7**	4.1	0.61
Trunk skinfolds	40.7**	5.6*	0.70
Extremity skinfolds	30.5**	6.9*	0.75
Trunk/extremity ratio	0.34	4.1	0.61
Sum skinfolds/total fat mass	0.72	6.7*	0.74

[a]An extra 4.2 mJ/day for 22 days in six pairs of MZ twins. Adapted from Poehlman et al., 1986. [b]The effects of overfeeding and the genotype-training interaction were assessed with a two-way analysis of variance for repeated measures on one factor. Intraclass coefficient computed with changes caused by overfeeding.
*$p < 0.05$; **$p < 0.01$.

tion of body fat stores as changes in energy balance (positive or negative) can alter total body fatness, although the sensitivity in the response will vary among individuals (Bouchard, Tremblay, et al., 1988; Poehlman et al., 1986). However, little is known about the variation in the response of various fat depots to changes in energy balance. From a theoretical point of view, as abdominal fat cells display a higher lipolytic response to catecholamines than femoral fat cells (Ostman, Arner, Engfeldt, & Kager, 1979; Rebuffé-Scrive et al., 1985; Smith, Hammersten, Björntorp, & Kral, 1979), it could be speculated that, in conditions of negative energy balance, lipid mobilization would be highest in the abdominal region.

In the Minnesota semistarvation study (Keys, Brozek, Henschel, Michelsen, & Taylor, 1950), the abdominal circumference was the anthropometric variable related to fatness that displayed the greatest reduction. Garn and Brozek (1956), however, have suggested that the amount of fat loss is proportional to the initial fat thickness before weight reduction. Therefore, it appears that the relative rate of fat loss does not display regional variation in response to a diet-induced energy deficit. Physiologically, however, it is important to keep in mind that the absolute amount of fat mobilized may be different among various adipose tissue regions and that this phenomenon could be the result of true metabolic differences among fat cells from different depots. After a 9-kg weight loss in obese women, Ashwell, Chinn, Stalley, and Garrow (1978) observed a greater reduction in waist diameter compared to thigh diameter, suggesting a greater mobilization of fat from the abdominal area. We must recognize, however, that very few studies have specifically addressed the issue of regional fat mobilization in response to a diet-induced negative energy balance (Himes, 1988) and that further studies using better methods are needed.

Exercise

In addition to low-calorie diets, an increase in energy expenditure due to regular aerobic exercise can produce a negative energy balance that can potentially induce a reduction in body fat stores. In men, we have shown that an aerobic exercise training program could significantly reduce body fat stores and that a caloric restriction was not necessary to induce a reduction in fat mass (Després et al., 1984; Tremblay, Després, Leblanc, & Bouchard, 1984). The response of various fat depots to physical training has not been extensively studied, however. As adipose tissue displays regional variation in its metabolic activity, it was of interest to study the effects of physical training on the mobilization of fat from different regions. We hypothesized that the abdominal depot, which has a high lipolytic activity (Ostman et al., 1979; Rebuffé-Scrive et al., 1985; Smith et al., 1979), should be more readily mobilized during aerobic exercise than peripheral depots. This hypothesis found some support in the observation of significant sex differences in the sensitivity to exercise training shown in Table 11.

Indeed, in nonobese individuals, we have consistently reported a reduction in fat mass following training for men but not for women (Després et al., 1984; Tremblay et al., 1984; Tremblay, Després, & Bouchard, 1988). As men have a greater accumulation of fat in the abdominal region than women, it is possible that the exercise-induced negative energy balance caused a greater mobilization of fat in men than in women. In an exercise program that induced in men a significant reduction in percent body fat, we have observed a greater mobilization of trunk skinfolds (27%) compared to extremity skinfolds (15%), suggesting a preferential mobilization of trunk fat (Table 12).

Tremblay et al. (1984) reported, in a sample of men subjected to an aerobic exercise training protocol, that the decrease in fat mass in response to training

Table 11

Effects of a 20-Week Aerobic Training Program on Body Fatness Variables in Men and Women

Variable (unit)	Before	After	T test
Women (N = 11)			
Body weight (kg)	54.2 ± 6.8	53.7 ± 7.2	n.s.
% Body fat	25.1 ± 5.2	22.0 ± 8.2	n.s.
Sum of 7 skinfolds (mm)	107.2 ± 25.3	113.0 ± 24.1	n.s.
Suprailiac fat cell weight (μg)	0.37 ± 0.11	0.34 ± 0.11	n.s.
Men (N = 11)			
Body weight (kg)	72.3 ± 16.3	69.4 ± 13.9	**
% Body fat	18.8 ± 9.4	15.6 ± 8.0	**
Sum of 7 skinfolds (mm)	103.0 ± 60.5	81.4 ± 42.5	**
Suprailiac fat cell weight (μg)	0.43 ± 0.15	0.37 ± 0.16	*

Note. Values are means ± *SD*. Adapted from Després et al., 1984.
*$p < 0.05$; **$p < 0.01$; n.s. = not significant.

Table 12

**Effect of a 15-Week High Intensity Exercise Training Program
on Body Fatness and Body Fat Distribution in Men**

Variable	Before training	After training	(% change)
Weight (kg)	63.8 ± 9.0	63.9 ± 9.3	n.s.
VO₂ (1/min)	2.93 ± 0.56	3.42 ± 0.61	(+17%)**
% Body fat	13.9 ± 4.8	11.2 ± 3.6	(−19%)*
Suprailiac fat cell diameter (μm)	84.4 ± 9.6	74.0 ± 11.3	(−17%)*
Trunk skinfolds (mm)	36.4 ± 9.5	26.6 ± 5.5	(−27%)**
Extremity skinfolds (mm)	26.9 ± 8.4	22.9 ± 5.7	(−15%)*
Ext/trunk	0.73 ± 0.05	0.86 ± 0.09	(+18%)**

Note. Values are means ± *SD*; n.s. = not significant. Trunk skinfolds = sum of subscapular, suprailiac, and abdominal skinfolds; Extremity skinfolds = sum of biceps, triceps, thigh, and calf skinfolds; Ext/trunk = extremity/trunk skinfolds ratio. Adapted from Després et al., 1988, and Tremblay et al., 1988.
*$p<0.05$; **$p<0.01$.

was proportional to the initial size of adipose cells obtained from the suprailiac depot, suggesting that abdominal fat cell hypertrophy could predict the loss of body fat in response to exercise. To further support such a model, Tremblay et al. (1984) divided their subjects on the basis of initial suprailiac fat cell size, as shown in Table 13. Men with low initial adipocyte size did not show any significant reduction in fat mass, whereas subjects with high initial fat cell size values displayed a mean reduction of fat mass reaching 4.2 kg after 20 weeks of aerobic training.

As we were not successful in reducing the adiposity of women by aerobic exercise training without controlling the caloric intake, it has not yet been possible to study regional fat mobilization in response to aerobic exercise training for women, and further research is needed in this area. However, results from our exercise training studies in men suggest a greater fat mobilization of subcutaneous trunk fat compared to peripheral fat. Additional studies using computed axial tomography will be needed to compare the mobilization of visceral fat to subcutaneous fat in response to aerobic exercise training.

As excess abdominal fat has been associated with numerous cardiovascular risk factors, one could ask whether the preferential mobilization of abdominal fat observed in men subjected to aerobic exercise could have beneficial effects on their metabolic profile. The potential associations between changes in adipose tissue distribution and changes in metabolic variables were studied in an experiment in which we subjected 12 young men to a 22-day aerobic exercise training program that induced a daily energy deficit of 4.2 MJ (Després, Moorjani, Tremblay, et al., 1988; Tremblay, Poehlman, Nadeau, Pérusse, & Bouchard, 1987). After training, subjects displayed a reduced plasma insulin response during an oral glucose challenge (Tremblay et al., 1987), which is a well-documented effect of exercise training (Björntorp, 1981).

Table 13

Influence of Initial Suprailiac Adipose Cell Size
on Exercise Training-Induced Fat Loss in Men

| | Initial adipose cell size | | |
Variable	High (*N* = 7)	Low (*N* = 7)	*T* test
Change in body weight (kg)	− 4.37 ± 4.71	0.13 ± 2.02	**
Change in fat mass (kg)	− 4.23 ± 3.78	− 0.70 ± 2.06	**
Change in sum of skinfolds (mm)	− 27.8 ± 21.7	− 7.2 ± 15.7	**

Note. Values are means ± *SD*. Adapted from Tremblay et al., 1984.
*$p < 0.05$; **$p < 0.01$.

Trained subjects also displayed reduced plasma triglyceride levels and an increase in the proportion of plasma cholesterol transported by high density lipoproteins. As shown in Table 14, the changes in plasma insulin and lipoprotein levels induced by exercise training, however, were totally dissociated from changes in maximal aerobic power and from changes in percent body fat, but were related to the proportion of trunk fat loss (Després, Moorjani, Tremblay, et al., 1988). Indeed, the higher the reduction in the proportion of trunk fat following training, the higher were the reductions in the plasma insulin response as well as in plasma cholesterol, LDL-cholesterol, and apoprotein B levels. Furthermore, a substantial reduction in the insulinogenic index (ratio of plasma insulin area/plasma glucose area during the glucose tolerance test) was associated with substantial decreases in plasma cholesterol, LDL-cholesterol, and apoprotein B levels. These results suggest that some of the beneficial effects of exercise training associated changes in fat distribution on plasma lipoprotein levels were mediated by changes in plasma insulin concentration. It therefore appears that the body fat distribution changes produced by exercise training can reduce the risk of cardiovascular disease by improving the metabolic profile of men.

Whether such an improvement can be observed in women subjected to aerobic exercise training will have to be studied, but we have reported that body fat distribution was an important variable to consider in assessing the effect of aerobic exercise training on the metabolic profile of obese women (Després, Tremblay, Nadeau, & Bouchard, 1988). Indeed, plasma glucose and insulin levels following a glucose challenge were measured in 34 obese premenopausal women before and after 6 months of aerobic training. Subjects exercised 90 minutes per day, 4 to 5 days a week, at an intensity varying from 65 to 75% of their maximal aerobic power.

As shown in Table 15, no significant change in body weight and body fat mass was noted after 6 months of training. Fasting plasma insulin levels as well as plasma insulin levels during the oral glucose tolerance test were significantly reduced after training. The response of plasma insulin levels to training, however, was associated with the initial level of body fat distribution. Indeed, women with a high waist-to-hip ratio and with high intra-abdominal fat accumulation (as

Table 14

Correlation Coefficients Between Relative Changes in $\dot{V}O_2$ max, % Body Fat, Body Fat Distribution, and Changes in Carbohydrate Metabolism and Plasma Lipoprotein Levels

	Relative changes in		
Relative changes in	$\dot{V}O_2$ max	% Body fat	Trunk/ext ratio
CHOL	−0.24	0.15	0.74**
TG	−0.05	−0.27	−0.19
Apo B	−0.15	0.28	0.72**
LDL-CHOL	−0.18	0.33	0.68*
HDL-CHOL	−0.04	0.14	0.40
Glucose area	0.00	−0.17	0.15
Insulin area	−0.09	−0.20	0.73**
Insulin/glucose areas	−0.12	−0.08	0.66*

Note. Adapted from Després et al., 1988; $N = 12$.
*$p < 0.05$; **$p < 0.01$; otherwise coefficients are not significant; CHOL = cholesterol; TG = triglycerides; Apo = apoprotein; LDL = low-density lipoprotein; HDL = high-density lipoprotein; Glucose area = sum of plasma glucose concentrations (mg/dl/180 min) during an oral glucose tolerance test; Insulin area = sum of plasma insulin concentrations (μU/ml/180 min) during the oral glucose tolerance test.

Table 15

Effects of a 6-Month Aerobic Exercise Training Program on Body Fatness and Plasma Glucose and Insulin Levels During an Oral Glucose Tolerance Test in Women With Low and High Abdominal Fat Accumulation

Variable (unit)	Before	After	p level
Women with low WHR[a] ($n = 10$)			
Weight (kg)	92.3 ± 18.5	92.4 ± 19.0	n.s.
% Body fat	48.9 ± 5.6	48.5 ± 5.4	n.s.
Glucose area (mg/dl/180m)	21,330 ± 5055	12,763 ± 5327	n.s.
Insulin area (μU/ml/180m)	13,294 ± 6962	12,763 ± 6195	n.s.
Women with high WHR[b] ($n = 10$)			
Weight (kg)	97.6 ± 16.0	95.3 ± 18.0	n.s.
% Body fat	47.9 ± 4.6	47.5 ± 6.6	n.s.
Glucose area (mg/dl/180m)	23,528 ± 3697	26,562 ± 9799	n.s.
Insulin area (μU/ml/180m)	16,964 ± 5348	13,172 ± 3236	<0.05

Note. Values are means ± SD; n.s. = not significant. Adapted from Després et al., 1988.
[a]Waist-to-hip circumferences ratio = 0.75 ± 0.04. [b]WHR = 0.87 ± 0.03.

measured by computed axial tomography) not only showed the highest plasma insulin concentrations during the glucose challenge but also displayed the greatest reduction in their plasma insulin concentration after glucose administration. Women with little intra-abdominal fat accumulation displayed a rather normal plasma insulin response that was not affected by training.

These results indicate, in concordance with the study by Krotkiewski and Björntorp (1986), that women with a high proportion of abdominal fat show high fasting plasma insulin levels and an exaggerated insulin response during a glucose challenge. But aerobic exercise training can improve their metabolic condition, although no reduction in body fat is observed. Exercise training experiments inducing fat loss in women are needed to verify whether a preferential mobilization of abdominal fat will have greater metabolic impacts than peripheral fat loss.

Changes in Body Fat Distribution During Fat Loss:
A Summary

In men, especially those who suffer from abdominal obesity, it seems that fat loss is associated with a preferential mobilization of trunk fat, although further studies with more sophisticated measures of body fat distribution are clearly needed. The metabolic impacts of diet-induced changes in body fat distribution are not known.

Exercise training per se can induce a reduction in fat mass in men, but resistance to exercise training-induced fat loss has been noted in women. In men, adipose tissue loss produced by aerobic exercise training appears to be greater in the trunk than in the extremities. It is not known whether this fat loss is associated with changes in the visceral/subcutaneous fat ratio. The magnitude of the trunk fat mobilization seems to determine the extent of the adaptation in the plasma insulin levels following exercise training. This body fat distribution-associated change in plasma insulin levels appears to play an important role in regulating the response of some plasma lipoproteins to exercise training. Finally, although it appears that obese women are resistant to exercise-induced fat loss, obese women with excess abdominal fat and metabolic complications benefit greatly from regular aerobic exercise.

IN SUMMARY

In elderly individuals, one can expect an increase of abdominal fat, particularly in the size of the visceral fat depot, even in the absence of an increase in total body fat. This phenomenon is of particular significance, as abdominal fat is a major risk factor for several metabolic complications and is associated with a higher death rate from cardiovascular diseases. Moreover, abdominal fat is now recognized as a risk factor independent of obesity per se. The relative risk of CHD-related deaths reaches about 1.5 in the obese while it attains about 2.0 in abdominal obesity.

Visceral fat increases as a result of positive energy balance, undetermined genetic characteristics, and elevated androgen production and sensitivity. However, with age, a positive energy balance may not even be a necessary condition, as shown by the data on fat redistribution in elderly individuals. Reduction in body fat requires a negative energy balance over a long period of time. It is still not entirely clear whether preferential abdominal fat mobilization can be achieved by dietary and/or exercise interventions. However, it has been suggested that if abdominal fat mobilization can be achieved, it would probably be more substantial in males than in females. One recent interesting finding is that improvement in the metabolic profile with regular exercise is more striking in the abdominal obese than in the peripheral obese. Therefore, due to its important clinical significance, the topic of abdominal fat in elderly people and its relationships to regular exercise and energy balance conditions should be carefully studied with better methods than those that have been generally used so far.

REFERENCES

ALBRINK, M.J., & Meigs, J.W. (1965). The relationship between serum triglycerides and skinfold thickness in obese subjects. *Annals of the New York Academy of Sciences,* **131**, 673-683.

ANDERSON, A.J., Sobocinski, K.A., Freedman, D.S., Barboriak, J.J., Rimm, A.A., & Gruchow, A.H. (1988). Body fat distribution, plasma lipids, and lipoproteins. *Arteriosclerosis,* **8**, 88-94.

ANDRES, R. (1985). Mortality and obesity: The rationale for age-specific height–weight tables. In R. Andres, E.L. Bierman, & W.R. Hazzard (Eds.), *Principles of geriatric medicine* (pp. 311-318). New York: McGraw-Hill.

ASHWELL, M., Chinn, S., Stalley, S., & Garrow, J.S. (1978). Female fat distribution—A photographic and cellularity study. *International Journal of Obesity,* **2**, 289-302.

ASHWELL, M., Cole, T.J., & Dixon, A.K. (1985). Obesity: New insight into the anthropometric classification of fat distribution by computed tomography. *British Medical Journal,* **290**, 1692-1694.

BJÖRNTORP, P. (1981). The effects of exercise on plasma insulin. *International Journal of Sports Medicine,* **2**, 125-129.

BJÖRNTORP, P. (1984). Hazards in subgroups of human obesity. *European Journal of Clinical Investigation,* **14**, 239-241.

BJÖRNTORP, P. (1985). Obesity and the risk of cardiovascular disease. *Annals of Clinical Research,* **17**, 3-9.

BLAIR, D., Habicht, J.P., Sims, E.A.H., Sylwester, D., & Abraham, S. (1984). Evidence for an increased risk for hypertension with centrally located body fat and the effect of race and sex on this risk. *American Journal of Epidemiology,* **119**, 526-540.

BOOTH, R.A.D., Goddard, B.A., & Paton, A. (1966). Measurement of fat thickness in man: A comparison of ultrasound, Harpenden calipers and electrical conductivity. *British Journal of Nutrition,* **20**, 719.

BORKAN, G.A., Gerzof, S.G., Robbins, A.H., Hults, D.E., Silbert, C.K., & Silbert, J.E. (1982). Assessment of abdominal fat content by computed tomography. *American Journal of Clinical Nutrition,* **36**, 172-177.

BORKAN, G.A., Hults, D.E., Gerzof, S.G., Robbins, A.H., & Silbert, C.K. (1983). Age changes in body composition revealed by computed tomography. *Journal of Gerontology,* **38**, 673-677.

BORKAN, G.A., & Norris, A.H. (1977). Fat redistribution and the changing body dimensions of the adult male. *Human Biology,* **49**, 495-514.

BOUCHARD, C. (1985). Inheritance of fat distribution and adipose tissue metabolism. In J. Vague, P. Björntorp, B. Guy-Grand, M. Rebuffé-Scrive, & P. Vague (Eds.), *Metabolic complications of human obesities* (pp. 87-96). Amsterdam: Elsevier.

BOUCHARD, C. (1987). Genetics of body fat, energy expenditure and adipose tissue metabolism. In E.M. Berry, S.H. Blondheim, H.E. Eliahou, & E. Shafrir (Eds.), *Recent advances in obesity research V* (pp. 16-25). London: John Libbey & Co.

BOUCHARD, C. (1988a). Gene–environment interaction in human adaptability. In R.M. Malina & H.M. Eckert (Eds.), *Physical activity in early and modern populations* (pp. 56-66). American Academy of Physical Education Papers, No. 21. Champaign, IL: Human Kinetics.

BOUCHARD, C. (1988b). Inheritance of human fat distribution. In C. Bouchard & F.E. Johnston (Eds.), *Fat distribution during growth and later health outcomes* (pp. 101-125). Current Topics in Nutrition and Disease, Vol. 17. New York: Alan R. Liss.

BOUCHARD, C. (1988c). Introductory notes on the topic of fat distribution. In C. Bouchard & F.E. Johnson (Eds.), *Fat distribution during growth and later health outcomes* (pp. 1-8). Current Topics in Nutrition and Disease, Vol. 17. New York: Alan R. Liss.

BOUCHARD, C. (1988). Genetic factors in the regulation of adipose tissue distribution. *Acta Medica Scandinavica* (Suppl. 723), 135-141.

BOUCHARD, C., & Johnston, F.E. (Eds.) (1988). *Fat distribution during growth and later health outcomes.* Current Topics in Nutrition and Disease, Vol. 17. New York: Alan R. Liss.

BOUCHARD, C., Pérusse, L., Leblanc, C., Tremblay, A., & Thériault, G. (1988). Heredity, human body fat and fat distribution. *International Journal of Obesity, 12*, 205-215.

BOUCHARD, C., Savard, R., Després, J.P., Tremblay, A., & Leblanc, C. (1985). Body composition in adopted and biological siblings. *Human Biology, 57*, 61-75.

BOUCHARD, C., Tremblay, A., Després, J.P., Poehlman, E.T., Thériault, G., Nadeau, A., Lupien, P., Moorjani, S., & Dussault, J. (1988). Sensitivity to overfeeding: The Quebec experiment with identical twins. *Progress in Food and Nutrition Science, 12*, 45-72.

CASTELLI, W.P. (1984). Epidemiology of coronary heart disease: The Framingham study. *American Journal of Medicine, 76*, 4-12.

CHRISTLIEB, A.R., Krolewski, A.S., Warram, J.H., & Soeldner, J.S. (1985). Is insulin the link between hypertension and obesity? *Hypertension, 7* (Suppl. 2), 54-57.

CLONINGER, C.R., Rice, J., & Reich, T. (1979). Multifactorial inheritance with cultural transmission and assortative mating. II. A general model of combined polygenic and cultural inheritance. *American Journal of Human Genetics, 31*, 176-198.

DeFRONZO, R.A. (1981). Insulin and renal sodium handling: Clinical implications. *International Journal of Obesity, 5* (Suppl. 1), 93-104.

DESPRÉS, J.P., Allard, C., Tremblay, A., Talbot, J., & Bouchard, C. (1985). Evidence for a regional component of body fatness in the association with serum lipids in men and women. *Metabolism, 34*, 967-973.

DESPRÉS, J.P., Bouchard, C., Savard, R., Tremblay, A., Marcotte, M., & Thériault, G. (1984). The effect of a 20-week endurance training program on adipose tissue morphology and lipolysis in men and women. *Metabolism, 33*, 235-239.

DESPRÉS, J.P., Bouchard, C., Tremblay, A., Savard, R., & Marcotte, M. (1985). Effects of aerobic training on fat distribution in male subjects. *Medicine and Science in Sports and Exercise,* **17,** 113-118.

DESPRÉS, J.P., Moorjani, S., Ferland, M., Tremblay, A., Lupien, P.J., Nadeau, A., Pinault, S., Thériault, G., & Bouchard, C. (1988). *Adipose tissue distribution and plasma lipoprotein levels in obese women: Importance of intra-abdominal fat.* Manuscript submitted for publication.

DESPRÉS, J.P., Moorjani, S., Tremblay, A., Poehlman, E.T., Lupien, P.J., Nadeau, A., & Bouchard, C. (1988). Heredity and changes in plasma lipids and lipoproteins following short-term exercise-training in men. *Arteriosclerosis,* **8,** 402-409.

DESPRÉS, J.P., Nadeau, A., Tremblay, A., Ferland, M., Moorjani, S., Lupien, P.J., Thériault, G., Pinault, S., & Bouchard, C. (1988). *Role of intra-abdominal fat in the association between regional adipose distribution and glucose tolerance in obese women.* Manuscript submitted for publication.

DESPRÉS, J.P., Tremblay, A., & Bouchard, C. (1988). Regional adipose tissue distribution and plasma lipoproteins. In C. Bouchard & F.E. Johnston (Eds.), *Fat distribution during growth and later health outcomes* (pp. 221-241). Current Topics in Nutrition and Disease, Vol. 17. New York: Alan R. Liss.

DESPRÉS, J.P., Tremblay, A., Nadeau, A., & Bouchard, C. (1988). Physical training and changes in regional adipose tissue distribution. *Acta Medica Scandinavica* (Suppl. 723), 205-212.

DESPRÉS, J.P., Tremblay, A., Pérusse, L., Leblanc, C., & Bouchard, C. (1988). Abdominal adipose tissue and serum HDL-cholesterol: Association independent from obesity and serum triglyceride concentration. *International Journal of Obesity,* **12,** 1-13.

DESPRÉS, J.P., Tremblay, A., Thériault, G., Pérusse, L., Leblanc, C., & Bouchard, C. (in press). Relationships between body fatness, adipose tissue distribution and blood pressure in men and women. *Journal of Clinical Epidemiology.*

ENZI, G., Gasparo, M., Biondetti, P.R., Fiore, D., Semisa, M., & Zurlo, F. (1986). Subcutaneous and visceral fat distribution according to sex, age, and overweight, evaluated by computed tomography. *American Journal of Clinical Nutrition,* **44,** 739-746.

EVANS, D.J., Hoffman, R.G., Kalkhoff, R.K., & Kissebah, A.H., (1984). Relationship of body fat topography to insulin sensitivity and metabolic profiles in premenopausal women. *Metabolism,* **33,** 68-75.

FEINLEIB, M. (1985). Epidemiology of obesity in relation to health hazards. *Annals of Internal Medicine,* **106,** 1019-1024.

FERLAND, M., Després, J.P., Tremblay, A., Pinault, S., Nadeau, A., Moorjani, S., Lupien, P.J., Thériault, G., & Bouchard, C. (1988). *Assessment of adipose tissue distribution by computed axial tomography in obese women: Association with body density and anthropometric measurements.* Manuscript submitted for publication.

FITNESS and Amateur Sport Canada. (1986). *Canadian Standardized Test of Fitness (CSTF). Operations manual* (3rd ed.). Ottawa: Government of Canada.

FOSTER, C.J., Wensier, R.L., Birch, R., Norris, D.J., Bernstein, R.S., Wang, J., Pierson, R.N., & Van Itallie, T.B. (1987). Obesity and serum lipids: An evaluation of the relative contribution of body fat and fat distribution to lipid levels. *International Journal of Obesity,* **11,** 151-162.

FUJIOKA, S., Matsuzawa, Y., Tokunaga, K., & Tarui, S. (1987). Contribution of intra-abdominal fat accumulation to the impairment of glucose and lipid metabolism in human obesity. *Metabolism, 36,* 54-59.

GARN, S.M., & Brozek, J. (1956). Fat changes during weight loss. *Science, 124,* 682.

GRAUER, W.O., Moss, A.A., Cann, C.E., & Goldberg, H.I. (1984). Quantification of body fat distribution in the abdomen using computed tomography. *American Journal of Clinical Nutrition, 39,* 631-637.

HAFFNER, S.M., Stern, M., Hazuda, H.P., Pugh, J., & Patterson, J.K. (1987). Do upper-body obesity and centralized adiposity measure different aspects of regional body-fat distribution? Relationship to non-insulin-dependent diabetes mellitus, lipids, and lipoproteins. *Diabetes, 36,* 43-51.

HARTZ, A.J., Rupley, D.C., Kalkhoff, R.D., & Rimm, A.A. (1983). Relationship of obesity to diabetes: Influence of obesity and fat distribution. *Preventive Medicine, 12,* 351-357.

HIMES, J.H. (1988). Alteration in distribution of adipose tissue in response to nutritional intervention. In C. Bouchard & F.E. Johnston (Eds.), *Fat distribution during growth and later health outcomes* (pp. 313-332). Current Topics in Nutrition and Disease, Vol. 17. New York: Alan R. Liss.

KALKHOFF, R.K., Hartz, A.H., Rupley, D., Kissebah, A.H., & Kelber, S. (1983). Relationship of body fat distribution to blood pressure, carbohydrate tolerance, and plasma lipids in healthy obese women. *Journal of Laboratory and Clinical Medicine, 102,* 621-627.

KEYS, A., Brozek, J., Henschel, A., Michelsen, F., & Taylor, H.L. (1950). *The biology of human starvation.* Minneapolis: University of Minnesota Press.

KISSEBAH, A.H., Evans, D.J., Peiris, A., & Wilson, C.R. (1985). Endocrine characteristics in regional obesities: Role of sex steroids. In J. Vague, P. Björntorp, B. Guy-Grand, M. Rebuffé-Scrive, & P. Vague (Eds.), *Metabolic complications of human obesities* (pp. 115-130). Amsterdam: Elsevier.

KISSEBAH, A.H., Peiris, A., & Evans, D.J. (1988). Mechanisms associating body fat distribution to glucose intolerance and diabetes mellitus. In C. Bouchard & F.E. Johnston (Eds.), *Fat distribution during growth and later health outcomes* (pp. 203-220). Current Topics in Nutrition and Disease, Vol. 17. New York: Alan R. Liss.,

KISSEBAH, A.H., Vydelingum, N., Murray, R., Evans, D.J., Hartz, A.J., Kalkhoff, R.K., & Adams, P.W. (1982). Relation of body fat distribution to metabolic complications of obesity. *Journal of Clinical Endocrinology and Metabolism, 54,* 254-260.

KROTKIEWSKI, M., & Björntorp, P. (1986). Muscle tissue in obesity with different distribution of adipose tissue. Effects of physical training. *European Journal of Applied Physiology, 10,* 331-341.

KROTKIEWSKI, M., Björntorp, P., Sjöström, L., & Smith, U. (1983). Impact of obesity on metabolism in men and women—Importance of regional adipose tissue distribution. *Journal of Clinical Investigation, 72,* 1150-1162.

KROTKIEWSKI, M., Mandroukas, K., Sjöström, L., Sullivan, L., Wetterqvist, H., & Björntorp, P. (1979). Effects of long-term physical training on body fat, metabolism, and blood pressure in obesity. *Metabolism, 28,* 650-658.

KVIST, H., Sjöström, L., & Tylen, U. (1986). Adipose tissue volume determinations in women by computed tomography. Technical considerations. *International Journal of Obesity,* **10**, 53-67.

LANDSBERG, L. (1986). Diet, obesity and hypertension: An hypothesis involving insulin, the sympathetic nervous system, and adaptive thermogenesis. *Quarterly Journal of Medicine,* **61**, 1081-1090.

MALINA, R.M., & Bouchard, C. (1988). Subcutaneous fat distribution during growth. In C. Bouchard & F.E. Johnston (Eds.), *Fat distribution during growth and later health outcomes* (pp. 63-84). Current Topics in Nutrition and Disease, Vol. 17. New York: Alan R. Liss.

NORGAN, N.G. (Ed.) (1985). *Human body composition and fat distribution.* (Report 8). Wageningen: Euro-Nut.

OHLSON, L.O., Larsson, B., Svärdsudd, K., Welin, L., Eriksson, H., Wilhemsen, L., Björntorp, P., & Tibblin, G. (1985). The influence of body fat distribution on the incidence of diabetes mellitus. 13.5 years of follow-up of the participants in the study of men born in 1913. *Diabetes,* **34**, 1055-1058.

OSLER, M. (1987). Obesity and cancer. *Danish Medical Bulletin,* **34**, 267-274.

OSTMAN, J., Arner, P., Engfeldt, P., & Kager, L. (1979). Regional differences in the control of lipolysis in human adipose tissue. *Metabolism,* **28**, 1198-1205.

PEIRIS, A., Mueller, R.A., Smith, G.A., Struve, M.F., & Kissebah, A.H. (1986). Splanchnic insulin metabolism in obesity: Influence of body fat distribution. *Journal of Clinical Investigation,* **78**, 1648-1657.

POEHLMAN, E.T., Tremblay, A., Després, J.P., Fontaine, E., Pérusse, L., Thériault, G., & Bouchard, C. (1986). Genotype-controlled changes in body composition and fat morphology following overfeeding in twins. *American Journal of Clinical Nutrition,* **43**, 723-731.

RABKIN, S.W., Mathewson, F.A.L., & Hsu, P.H. (1977). Relation of body weight to development of ischemic heart disease in a cohort of young North American men after a 26-year observation period: The Manitoba study. *American Journal of Cardiology,* **39**, 452-458.

REBUFFÉ-SCRIVE, M., Enk, L., Crona, N., Lönnroth, P., Abrahamsson, L., Smith, U., & Björntorp, P. (1985). Fat cell metabolism in different regions in women. Effects of menstrual cycle, pregnancy, and lactation. *Journal of Clinical Investigation,* **75**, 1973-1976.

SEIDELL, J.C., Oosterlee, A., Thyssen, M.A.O., Burema, J., Deurenberg, P., Hautvast, J.G.A.G., & Ruys, J.H.J. (1987). Assessment of intra-abdominal and subcutaneous abdominal fat: Relation between anthropometry and computed tomography. *American Journal of Clinical Nutrition,* **45**, 7-13.

SIMOPOULOS, A.P., & Van Italie, T. (1984). Body weight, health and longevity. *Annals of Internal Medicine,* **100**, 285-295.

SIMS, E.A.H., & Berchtold, P. (1982). Obesity and hypertension: Mechanisms and implications for management. *Journal of the American Medical Association,* **247**, 49-52.

SJÖSTRÖM, L. (1988). Measurement of fat distribution. In C. Bouchard & F.E. Johnston (Eds.), *Fat distribution during growth and later health outcomes* (pp. 43-61). Current Topics in Nutrition and Disease, Vol. 17. New York: Alan R. Liss.

SJÖSTRÖM, L., Kvist, H., Cederblad, A., & Tylen, U. (1986). Determination of the total adipose tissue volume in women by computed tomography. Comparisons with ^{40}K and tritium techniques. *American Journal of Physiology*, **250**, E736-E745.

SJÖSTRÖM, L., Kvist, H., & Tylen, U. (1985). Methodological aspects of measurements of adipose tissue distribution. In J. Vague, P. Björntorp, B. Guy-Grand, M. Rebuffé-Scrive, & P. Vague (Eds.), *Metabolic complications of human obesities* (pp. 13-19). Amsterdam: Elsevier.

SMITH, U., Hammersten, J., Björntorp, P., & Kral, J.G. (1979). Regional differences and effect of weight reduction on human fat cell metabolism. *European Journal of Clinical Investigation*, **9**, 327-332.

SPARROW, D., Borkan, G.A., Gerzof, S.G., Wisniewski, C., & Silbert, C.K. (1986). Relationship of body fat distribution to glucose tolerance. Results of computed tomography in male participants of the normative aging study. *Diabetes*, **35**, 411-415.

TERRY, R.B., Stefanick, M.L., Krauss, R.M., Haskell, W.L., & Wood, P.D. (1985). Relationships between abdomen to hip ratio, plasma lipoproteins and sex hormones. *Circulation*, **72**, 452A.

TOKUNAGA, K., Matsuzawa, Y., Ishikawa, K., & Tarui, S. (1983). A novel technique for the determination of body fat by computed tomography. *International Journal of Obesity*, **7**, 437-445.

TREMBLAY, A., Després, J.P., & Bouchard, C. (1988). Alteration in body fat and fat distribution with exercise. In C. Bouchard & F.E. Johnston (Eds.), *Fat distribution during growth and later health outcomes* (pp. 297-312). Current Topics in Nutrition and Disease, Vol. 17. New York: Alan R. Liss.

TREMBLAY, A., Després, J.P., Leblanc, C., & Bouchard, C. (1984). Sex dimorphism in fat loss in response to exercise-training. *Journal of Obesity and Weight Regulation*, **3**, 193-203.

TREMBLAY, A., Poehlman, E.T., Nadeau, A., Pérusse, L., & Bouchard, C. (1987). Is the response of plasma glucose and insulin to short-term exercise-training genetically determined? *Hormone and Metabolic Research*, **19**, 65-67.

VAGUE, J. (1947). Les obésités. Étude biométrique [Obesities: Biometric studies]. *Biologie Médicale*, **36**, 1-47.

VAGUE, J. (1956). The degree of masculine differentiation of obesities: A factor determining predisposition to diabetes, gout and uric calculous disease. *American Journal of Clinical Nutrition*, **4**, 20-34.

VAGUE, J., Björntorp, P., Guy-Grand, B., Rebuffé-Scrive, M., & Vague, P. (F
(1985). *Metabolic complications of human obesities*. Amsterdam: Elsevier.

WEINSIER, R.L., Norris, D.J., Birch, R., Bernstein, R.S., Wang, J., Y
Pierson, R.N., & Van Itallie, T.B. (1985). The relative contribution of '
pattern to blood pressure level. *Hypertension*, **7**, 578-585.

Acknowledgments

The studies from the authors' laboratory were supported by the Natural Sciences and Engineering Research Council of Canada (G-0850, A-8150, and A-3609), FCAR-Québec (EQ-1330), Canadian Fitness and Lifestyle Research Institute (8605-2446-1048), Canadian Heart Foundation, Health and Welfare Canada (6605-2769-56), and the National Institutes of Health (R01DK34624). Jean-Pierre Després is a research scholar from the FRSQ-Québec. Thanks are expressed to Drs. Angelo Tremblay, Germain Thériault, Eric T. Poehlman, Louis Pérusse, André Nadeau, Sital Moorjani, Paul Lupien, and other colleagues from the Physical Activity Sciences Laboratory and the Department of Medicine who were involved in these studies.

Osteoporosis, Bone Mineral, and Exercise

Everett L. Smith and Catherine Gilligan
University of Wisconsin–Madison

Bone tissue consists primarily of inorganic mineral crystalline structures (composed primarily of calcium and phosphorus) and organic components (primarily collagen). There are two forms of bone tissue: compact and cancellous bone. Compact, or cortical bone, consists of tightly packed layers of mineralized structure supplied with nutrients from capillaries and comprises the major portions of the long bones. Cancellous bone comprises the major portions of the vertebrae and the ends of the long bones. Ninety-nine percent of the calcium in the human body is contained in the skeletal structure.

The body has three types of bone cells: osteocytes (bone maintenance), osteoblasts (bone formation), and osteoclasts (bone resorption). In the adult, osteoblasts and osteoclasts are generally coupled and work in conjunction with each other in bone remodeling. The osteoclasts remove bone, and the resorption spaces are subsequently filled by osteoblasts in two stages (matrix synthesis followed by mineralization). The new bone matrix, called the osteoid seam, is circular in cortical bone and crescent-shaped in cancellous bone. The volume of bone formed depends on the number of osteoblasts assembled as a result of the formation stimuli, whether biomechanical or hormonal. Bone turnover starts with osteoclastic activation on a quiescent surface and ends after the osteoblast formation activity is complete and the bone surface is once more quiescent. Activation seems to occur partly at random and partly in response to mechanical strain (Parfitt, 1987).

It has commonly been accepted that the composition and general characteristics of osteoporotic bone are identical to those of normal bone with the only difference being quantity. Ferris, Klenerman, Dodds, Bitensky, and Chayen (1987), however, indicated that both the quality and quantity of the bone may be affected in osteoporosis. The quantity of bone or bone mineral content (BMC) is highly correlated with bone strength (0.90) and is often used as an indicator of bone strength.

In addition to bone mineral mass, however, other factors in bone quality, such as bone geometry, collagen orientation, and bone composition, contribute to bone strength. At present, the effect of aging, disuse, and physical activity on these factors is ill-defined. Histomorphometry can be used to evaluate the effect of various factors on bone geometry. Tetracycline labeling allows the evaluation of the location and rate of bone cell activity in response to interventions.

Tetracycline binds to calcium and is incorporated into the bone during mineralization, and therefore is useful as an event marker in the study of bone modeling and remodeling. The incorporation of tetracycline in mineral marks the site of bone formation and provides formation rates when double labels are used. Lanyon (1984) presented histologic evidence that osteoblastic (formation) and osteoclastic (resorption) activities are affected by mechanical strain level and number of cycles.

Bone functions primarily as mechanical support and as a mineral storehouse. Correspondingly, bone resorption and formation are responsive both to mechanical forces and to hormones regulating calcium homeostasis. Increased mechanical loads (such as exercise) call for increased bone mass, and decreased mechanical loads (such as bed rest) cause bone atrophy as the unneeded mass is resorbed. Dietary deficiencies, through a complex hormonal system, increase net bone resorption. Estrogen deficiency at menopause also produces a greater net bone resorption, partly through its effect on calcium metabolism.

OSTEOPOROSIS

Osteoporosis, the result of excessive bone loss, is defined as the presence of fractures with little or no contributing trauma. As the population ages, so does the prevalence of osteoporosis. Both women and men lose bone mass with age, but the loss in women starts earlier and proceeds at a greater rate. Osteoporosis occurs most often as fractures of the hip, spine (compression or wedging fractures), and wrist (Colles' fractures). Approximately 1.3 million osteoporotic fractures occur annually in the U.S., at a cost of $3.8 billion (NIH, 1984).

The etiology of bone loss with age is multifactorial. Factors include heredity, peak bone mass at maturity, postmenopausal status (estrogen depletion), chronological age, inadequate calcium intake or malabsorption, decreased physical activity, and lifestyle. The most prominent factor in women is estrogen deficiency following menopause, which accelerates bone loss. The mechanism by which estrogen deficiency contributes to bone loss is unknown. Calcium metabolism appears to be affected by menopause, as fractional calcium absorption decreases with the change from premenopausal to postmenopausal status (Heaney, Recker, & Saville, 1978). Dietary calcium insufficiency is another suspected factor in the etiology of osteoporosis, although evidence regarding the effect of calcium intake on bone mass or bone loss rates is mixed. Calcium absorption decreases with age, and calcium malabsorption is more common in osteoporotics than normal subjects of the same age (Gallagher et al., 1979; Nordin et al., 1976). Other risk factors include low peak adult bone mass, being of northern European origin, having a small skeletal frame or low body weight, and certain disease states.

Lifestyle factors such as smoking, alcohol consumption, and nutrition factors other than calcium may also contribute to bone loss and increase the risk of osteoporosis (Freudenheim, Johnson, & Smith, 1986). One important factor frequently overlooked in the etiology of osteoporosis is hypokinesis. Most people tend to exercise less, and their general fitness decreases as they age. As shown in studies of bed rest, decreased activity promotes bone loss.

There are three modes most commonly considered in the prevention of osteoporosis; estrogen replacement therapy for postmenopausal women, calcium supplementation, and increased physical activity. Although estrogen replacement therapy halts bone loss, many are concerned about its possible side effects. Calcium supplementation is currently controversial, as few studies show an indisputable effect of calcium on bone loss. Studies have shown, however, that a postmenopausal estrogen-deplete woman requires 1,500 mg calcium/day to maintain calcium balance (Heaney et al., 1978). Physical activity, while it has shown promise in counteracting or even reversing bone loss, needs further investigation to determine the optimal modes and levels of activity for the group at risk.

Once osteoporotic fractures of the spine are incurred, little can be done to repair the damage to the bone. Attempts to prevent further fractures have included the three preventive methods listed above, as well as fluoride, PTH, calcitonin, and vitamin D therapies.

Physical Activity and Osteoporosis

The effect of mechanical forces on bone is most evident in extreme states such as weightlessness, bed rest, and vigorous athletic training. In weightlessness and bed rest, bone mineral content of the spine and calcaneous decrease by about 1% per week. Athletes have bone mineral content up to 35% greater than average. These activity levels, however, reflect neither the normal activity of the population at risk (postmenopausal women) nor a level of activity that is reasonable for the average women to pursue for a lifetime. Cross-sectional studies of bone mass in ambulatory nonathletes have not shown as prominent an effect of physical activity on bone as have studies of athletes. However, intervention studies have demonstrated that bone loss can be prevented or reversed by physical training even in postmenopausal, osteoporotic, and elderly women.

Induced Osteoporosis by Weightlessness or Bed Rest

The removal or decrease of muscular or gravitational forces on bone segments causes bone atrophy. The degree of atrophy is influenced by the typical strains on the bone segment, with segments normally required to carry a greater load showing a more rapid atrophy when loads are decreased or removed.

Most studies of astronauts have measured response of the os calcis and forearm to weightlessness. Os calcis loss, measured by single photon absorptiometry, was approximately 0.1% per day in flights of 10 to 185 days (Rambaut, Smith, Mack, & Vogel, 1975; Smith, Rambaut, Vogel, & Whittle, 1977; Stupakov, Kazaykin, Kozlovsky, & Korolev, 1984; Tilton, Degioanni, & Schneider, 1980; Vogel, 1975; Vogel & Whittle, 1976). Radius and ulna bone mineral content, however, was not significantly affected (Rambaut, Smith, et al., 1975; Smith et al., 1977; Tilton et al., 1980; Vogel, 1975; Vogel & Whittle, 1976). The losses in bone were paralleled by changes in calcium metabolism. Calcium balance declined while both urinary and fecel excretion of calcium increased (Biriukov & Krasnykh, 1970; Brodzinski, Rancitelli, Haller, & Dewey, 1971; Leach & Rambaut, 1975; Lutwak, Whedon, LaChance, Reid, & Lipscomb, 1969; Rambaut, Leach, & Johnson, 1975; Whedon et al., 1974). Urinary hydroxyproline, a measure of bone resorption, increased in the Skylab studies (Leach & Rambaut, 1975; Leach, Rambaut, & DeFerranti, 1979; Whedon et al., 1974). It is uncertain whether loss tapers off with longer spaceflights. While it is hypothesized that spaceflight affects bone mass primarily in the habitually weight-bearing bones, the effects of weightlessness on the tibia, femur, and spine have not been determined.

Bed rest mimics weightlessness by changing the vectors of gravitational forces acting on the weight-bearing bones. As in weightlessness, calcium balance declines with bed rest (Deitrick, Whedon, & Shorr, 1948; Donaldson et al., 1970; Goldsmith, Killian, Ingbar, & Bass, 1969; Hulley et al., 1971; Schneider & McDonald, 1984). In these studies, calcium balance began to increase after approximately 7 weeks but remained depressed from normal levels even after 36 weeks (Schneider & McDonald, 1984). The greatest changes in bone mineral content during bed rest occurred in trabecular weight-bearing bones such as the os calcis and lumbar spine (Hansson, Roos, & Nachemson, 1975; Hulley et al., 1971; Krolner & Toft, 1983; Schneider & McDonald, 1984), with little demineralization of the upper extremities (Hulley et al., 1971; Whedon, 1984). Attempts to counter bed-rest-induced bone loss in healthy normal subjects by non-weight-bearing activity have met with limited success. Supine or seated exercise, intermittent longitudinal compression, hydrostatic pressure, and sitting all failed to reverse the calcium lost with bed rest (Hantman et al., 1973; Issekutz, Blizzard, Birkhead, & Rodahl, 1966; Ragan & Briscoe, 1964; Schneider & McDonald, 1984). Quiet standing, however, appeared to prevent bone loss and improve calcium (Issekutz et al., 1966).

PREVENTION OF BONE LOSS BY PHYSICAL ACTIVITY

A number of researchers have reported that bone mass of the weight-bearing (femur, spine, calcaneous, tibia) and non-weight-bearing (radius, ulna, humerus) bones are higher in athletes than in matched sedentary controls (Aloia, Cohn, Babu, et al., 1978; Brewer, Meyer, Keele, Upton, & Hagan, 1983; Dalen & Olsson, 1974; Lane et al., 1986). The location and degree of hypertrophy are influenced by the specific sport; for example, femur and spine bone density were highest in weightlifters and lowest in swimmers (Block, Genant, & Black, 1986; Jacobson, Beaver, Grubb, Taft, & Talmage, 1984; Nilsson & Westlin, 1971). Evidence that higher bone mass is not entirely due to the heredity of athletes is provided by studies of tennis and baseball players. Both male and female participants in these unilateral sports have pronounced bone hypertrophy in the dominant arm despite normal values in the nondominant arm (Jacobson, Beaver, Janeway, et al., 1984; Jones, Priest, & Hayes, 1977; Priest, Jones, Tichnor, & Nagel, 1977; Watson, 1974). Bone hypertrophy in response to activity does not appear to be limited by age, as it has been observed in elderly (ages 60–84) tennis players as well as in the young (Huddleston, Rockwell, Kulund, & Harrison, 1980; Montoye, Smith, Fardon, & Howley, 1980).

Most cross-sectional studies of nonathletes have reported that the correlation of physical activity with bone mass is poor (Aloia, Vaswani, Yeh, & Cohn, 1988; Black-Sandler et al., 1982; Emiola & O'Shea, 1978; Frisancho, Montoye, Frantz, Metzner, & Dodge, 1970; Kanders, Dempster, & Lindsay, 1988; Krolner, Tondevold, Toft, Berthelson, & Nielsen, 1982; Maini, Lamba, & Singh, 1980; Montoye, McCabe, Metzner, & Garn, 1976; Oyster, Morton, & Linnell, 1984; Stillman, Lohman, Slaughter, & Massey, 1986; Yano, Wasnich, Vogel, & Heilbrun, 1984; Zanzi, Ellis, Aloia, & Cohn, 1981). This may be due to the narrow range of physical activity levels in the average populace, difficulties in measurement and quantification of physical activity levels and types, and selection of bone sites not affected by the subjects' activities. Some studies reported that bone mass was greater in high-activity groups than low- or moderate-activity groups, but that low- and moderate-activity groups did not differ in bone mass of the second phalange or radius (Emiola & O'Shea, 1978; Stillman et al., 1986).

Black-Sandler et al. (1982) provided an example of how variation in methods of evaluating physical activity may affect the interpretation of the relationship between physical activity and bone. They found that radius and tibial bone mass were related to physical activity level measured by activity monitors, but not by interview. For the weight-bearing bones—spine, femur, and os calcis—bone mass was correlated with physical activity level in most (Aloia et al., 1988; Jacobson, Beaver, Janeway, et al., 1984; Kanders et al., 1988; Krolner et al., 1982; Maini et al., 1980; Yano et al., 1984) but not all studies (Lindquist, Bengtsson, Hansson, & Roos, 1979; Zanzi et al., 1981).

Conversely, the association of physical activity level to bone mass in the non-weight-bearing bones of the forearm—metacarpal, radius, ulna—was typically nonsignificant (Aloia et al., 1988; Kanders et al., 1988; Krolner et al., 1982; Montoye, 1975; Montoye et al., 1976; Yano et al., 1984; Zanzi et al., 1981). However, several studies (Anderson & Halioua, 1986; Ballard, McKeouwn, Graham, Milner, & Zinkgraf, 1986; Halioua, 1986; Jacobson, Beaver, Grubb, et al., 1984; Oyster et al., 1984) reported that women with high activity levels had greater radius BMC or metacarpal cortical diameter than women with low activity levels. It should be noted that the active group in Jacobson's study consisted of women who played tennis regularly.

The correlation of fitness level to bone mass appears to be stronger than that of physical activity level. Again, the greater association occurs with weight-bearing bones, and a lesser or nonsignificant correlation with non-weight-bearing bones of the arm (Chow, Harrison, Brown, & Hajek, 1986; Krolner et al., 1982; Montoye et al., 1976; Pocock et al., 1987; Pocock, Eisman, Yeates, Sambrook, & Eberl, 1986). The association between aerobic work capacity and bone is indirect, and probably due in each case to the influence of physical activities. Other studies have reported that local and total bone mass and muscle mass or strength are correlated for the spine and total body calcium (Doyle, Brown, & LaChance, 1970; Harrison, 1984; Pocock et al., 1987; Sinaki, McPhee, Hodgson, Merritt, & Offord, 1986; Sinaki, Opitz, & Wahner, 1974; Zanzi et al., 1980). Either grip or elbow flexor strength was correlated with bone mass in one study (Pocock et al., 1987) but not another (Sinaki et al., 1974). Total body potassium and the ratio of left psoas width to L3 width were lower in osteoporotic subjects than in control subjects (Ellis, Shukla, Cohn, & Pierson, 1974; Pogrund, Bloom, & Weinberg, 1986).

In most studies in which formerly sedentary subjects participated in a regular physical activity program, bone hypertrophied or bone loss was decreased compared to controls. The reported effect of physical activity intervention on bone may be modulated by the type and intensity of the activities, the bone sites evaluated, and the subject population. Dalen and Olsson (1974) studied 19 men (ages 25–52) who walked or ran 15 km/week for 3 months. The training regimen did not significantly affect BMC of the seven axial and appendicular sites measured. Similarly, men training an average of 65 km/month for a marathon did not significantly change in os calcis BMC (Williams, Wagner, Wasnich, & Heilbrun, 1984). However, more consistent runners (141 km/month) in the same study increased significantly (3%) in os calcis BMC.

Overton, Hangartner, Heath, and Ridley (1981) reported that distal radius bone density in three young male athletes increased 1–4% during 1–4 months of weight training for arm strength. A very rigorous training program (8 hours/day, 6 days/week) produced greater bone hypertrophy than these less intense programs (Margulies et al., 1986). Tibial, BMC increased 8–12% in 158 male military recruits, ages 18–21, who completed the 14-week regimen. Hypertrophy was less pronounced (1–9%) in 110 subjects who discontinued training because of injury (primarily fractures).

The most common target group for studying physical activity intervention effects on bone is postmenopausal women, whose average rate of loss predisposes them to osteoporosis. Aloia, Cohn, Ostuni, Cane, and Ellis (1978) found that total body calcium, but not radius BMC, improved significantly relative to controls ($n=9$) in nine postmenopausal women who exercised three times/week for a year. The training program consisted primarily of aerobic, weight-bearing activities with no special emphasis on the arms. Sandler et al. (1984) also reported that radius BMC change did not differ between women who increased their walking by 68% and those who increased by 28%. These training regimens and the difference between groups were modest, and also did not place much additional stress on the arms. In contrast, White, Martin, Yeater, Butcher, and Radin (1984) found that radius BMC declined significantly in 6 months in both control ($n=21$) and walking ($n=27$; 1–2 miles, 2–4 times/week) groups, but did not change significantly in an aerobic dance group ($n=25$; 2–5 dances, 2–4 times/week). The authors hypothesized that the arm movements during aerobic dance deterred bone loss in the radius.

Several investigators have designed training programs that incorporate both aerobic weight-bearing and upper body strengthening activities. Smith, Gilligan, Shea, Ensign, and Smith (in preparation) reported that bone loss of the radius and ulna was significantly reduced in 80 women (ages 35–65) exercising 45 minutes/session, three times/week for 4 years relative to 62 control subjects. Humerus bone loss also tended to be lower in the exercise subjects. Chow, Harrison, and Notarius (1987) divided 48 postmenopausal women (ages 50–59) into three groups: control, aerobic exercise, and aerobic plus strength exercise. The two intervention groups trained 1 hour, three times/week for a year. The calcium bone index (CABI, total calcium of the trunk and upper thighs adjusted for body size) did not change significantly in any group, although it tended to increase in exercise groups and decrease in the control group. The amount of change differed significantly between the control and exercise groups, but the two training regimens did not differ significantly in their effect on CABI.

Dalsky et al. (1988) studied 33 postmenopausal women ages 55 to 70:17 exercise subjects and 16 controls. The training sessions consisted of 30–40 minutes of aerobic weight-bearing activity and 15–20 minutes of upper body work and were held three times/week. Integral BMC of the spine (L2–L4) increased 5.2% with 9 months' training ($n=17$) and 6.1% with 22 months' training ($n=11$), while it decreased 1.4% and 1.1% in control subjects followed for the same time periods. BMC declined 4.8% in 13 months of detraining for 15 of the trained subjects.

Another important question is whether bone loss can be averted or reversed in women who have already experienced osteoporotic fractures. Krolner, Toft, Nielson, and Tondevold (1983) studied the effects of 8 months' exercise training for 1 hour, twice/week on women with recent Colles' fractures (ages 50–73).

Lumbar spine BMC increased 3.5% in the exercise group, which was significantly different from the control group loss of 2.7%. Change in forearm BMC did not differ significantly between age groups. Similar to the study of Aloia, Cohn, Ostuni, et al. (1978), the primary mode of training was aerobic weight-bearing activity.

In contrast, Simkin and colleagues (Ayalon, Simkin, Leichter, & Raifmann, 1987; Simkin, Ayalon, & Leichter, 1986) combined 15 minutes of dynamic loading to the forearm with 30 minutes of aerobic movement, warm-up, stretching, and relaxation in sessions meeting three times/week for 5 months. The subjects were classified as osteoporotic on the basis of morphological changes in the spine. Distal radius BMC (measured by SPA) and trabecular mass density (MD, measured by Compton scattering) were evaluated during a 1-year nonintervention period and the 5-month intervention period. MD decreased significantly in both the exercise (2.0%, $n=14$) and control (2.8%, $n=26$) groups during the observation period, and continued to decline in the control group during the 5-month treatment period (1.9%), but increased significantly with training in the exercise subjects (3.8%). BMC, however, did not change significantly in either group.

Chow, Harrison, Sturtbridge, et al. (1987) also incorporated both strength training (20 min.) and aerobic exercise (30 min.) in a 12.5-month study of osteoporotic women concurrently receiving fluoride treatment. All subjects were instructed to follow the training regimen. Subjects who exercised regularly ($n=20$, at least three times/week) had a significantly greater CABI at the end of the study (17% increase) than the subjects who did not train ($n=15$) or who trained two or fewer times per week ($n=3$) (6% increase). The authors attributed the increase in the nontraining group to the fluoride treatment.

Only a few studies have addressed the effect of physical activity intervention on bone in the elderly. Smith, Reddan, and Smith (1981) conducted a 3-year study of women (*M* age 81) in a nursing home. Twelve subjects participated 3 times/week in a low-intensity program of chair exercises, and 18 subjects served as controls. The control group exhibited a significant decline in radius BMC (-3.3%) while that of the exercise group did not change significantly ($+2.3\%$). The change in both radius BMC and BMC/W differed significantly between groups. Rundgren, Aniansson, Ljungberg, and Wetterquist (1984) reported that after a 9-month training program held twice/week for 1 hour, 15 elderly women (*M* age 72) had significantly greater heel BMC than did control subjects, although there was no significant change in the training subjects. Sidney, Shephard, and Harrison (1977) reported that total body calcium did not change significantly in 14 elderly men and women exercising four times/week for a year.

The common decrease in physical activity with age may contribute to bone loss, as suggested by studies on bed rest and weightlessness. Conversely, studies on athletes and formerly sedentary subjects who increase their physical activity show that exercise promotes bone hypertrophy and counteracts bone loss.

REFERENCES

ALOIA, J.F., Cohn, S.H., Babu, T., Abesamis, C., Kalici, N., & Ellis, K. (1978). Skeletal mass and body composition in marathon runners. *Metabolism, 27*, 1793.

ALOIA, J.F., Cohn, S.H., Ostuni, J., Cane, R., & Ellis, K. (1978). Prevention of involutional bone loss by exercise. *Annals of Internal Medicine, 89*, 356-358.

ALOIA, J.F., Vaswani, A.N., Yeh, J.K., & Cohn, S.H. (1988). Premenopausal bone mass is related to physical activity. *Archives of Internal Medicine, 148*(1), 121-123.

ANDERSON, J.J.B., & Halioua, L. (1986). Combined effects of past physical activity (PA) and calcium (Ca) intake on current radial bone parameters in premenopausal women. *Federation Proceedings, 45*, 594.

AYALON, J., Simkin, A., Leichter, I., & Raifmann, S. (1987). Dynamic bone loading exercises for postmenopausal women: Effect on the density of the distal radius. *Archives of Physical Medicine and Rehabilitation, 68*, 280-283.

BALLARD, J., McKeouwn, B., Graham, H., Milner, A., & Zinkgraf, S. (1986). The effect of physical activity and estrogen therapy upon bone loss in postmenopausal females, aged 50-68 years. *Medicine and Science in Sports and Exercise, 18*, 520.

BIRIUKOV, E.N., & Krasnykh, I.G. (1970). Changes in the optical density of bone tissue and in the calcium metabolism of the cosmonauts. *Kosm Biol Med, 4*, 42-45.

BLACK-SANDLER, R., LaPorte, R.E., Sashin, D., Kuller, L.H., Sternglass, E., Cauley, J.A., & Link, M.M. (1982). Determinants of bone mass in menopause. *Preventive Medicine, 11*, 269-280.

BLOCK, J.E., Genant, H.K., & Black, D. (1986). Greater vertebral bone mineral mass in exercising young men. *Western Journal of Medicine, 145*, 39-42.

BREWER, V., Meyer, B.M., Keele, M.S., Upton, S.J., & Hagan, R.D. (1983). Role of exercise in prevention of involutional bone loss. *Medicine and Science in Sports and Exercise, 15*, 445-449.

BRODZINSKI, R.L., Rancitelli, L.A., Haller, W.A., & Dewey, L.S. (1971). Calcium, potassium and iron loss by Apollo 7, 8, 9, 10 and 11 astronauts. *Aerospace Medicine, 42*, 621-626.

CHOW, R.K., Harrison, J.E., Brown, C.F., & Hajek, V. (1986). Physical fitness effect on bone mass in postmenopausal women. *Archives of Physical Medicine and Rehabilitation, 67*, 231-234.

CHOW, R.K., Harrison, J.E., & Notarius, C. (1987). Effect of two randomized exercise programmes on bone mass of healthy postmenopausal women. *British Medical Journal, 292*, 607-610.

CHOW, R.K., Harrison, J.E., Sturtbridge, W., Josse, R., Murray, T.M., Bayley, A., Dornan, J., & Hammond, T. (1987). The effect of exercise on bone mass of osteoporotic patients on fluoride treatment. *Clinical and Investigative Medicine, 10*, 59-63.

DALEN, N., & Olsson, K.E. (1974). Bone mineral content and physical activity. *Acta Orthopedica Scandinavica, 45*, 170-174.

DALSKY, G.P., Stocke, K.S., Ehsani, A.A., Slatopolsky, E., Lee, W.C.P., & Birge, S.J. (1988). Weight-bearing exercise training and lumbar bone mineral content in postmenopausal women. *Annals of Internal Medicine, 108*, 824-828.

DEITRICK, J.E., Whedon, G.D., & Shorr, E. (1948). Effects of immobilization upon various metabolic and physiologic functions of normal men. *American Journal of Medicine, 4*, 3-35.

DONALDSON, C.L., Hulley, S.B., Vogel, J.M., Hattner, R.S., Bayers, J.H., & McMillan, D.E. (1970). Effect of prolonged bed rest on bone mineral. *Metabolism, 19*, 1071-1084.

DOYLE, F., Brown, J., & LaChance, C. (1970, February 21). Relation between bone mass and muscle weight. *Lancet,* pp. 391-393.

ELLIS, K.J., Shukla, K.K., Cohn, S.H., & Pierson, R.N. (1974). A predictor for total body potassium in man based on height, weight, sex and age: Applications in metabolic disorders. *Journal of Laboratory and Clinical Medicine,* **83**, 716-727.

EMIOLA, L., & O'Shea, P. (1978). Effects of physical activity and nutrition on bone density measured by radiographic techniques. *Nutrition Reports International,* **17**(6), 669-681.

FERRIS, B.D., Klenerman, L., Dodds, R.A., Bitensky, L., & Chayen, J. (1987). Altered organization of non-collagenous bone matrix in osteoporosis. *Bone,* **8**(5), 285-288.

FREUDENHEIM, J.L., Johnson, N.E., & Smith, E.L. (1986). Relationships between usual nutrient intake and bone-mineral content of women 35–65 years of age: Longitudinal and cross-sectional analysis. *American Journal of Clinical Nutrition,* **44**, 683-676.

FRISANCHO, A.R., Montoye, H.J., Frantz, M.E., Metzner, H., & Dodge, H.J. (1970). A comparison of morphological variables in adult males selected on the basis of physical activity. *Medicine and Science in Sports,* **2**, 209-212.

GALLAGHER, J.C., Riggs, B.L., Eisman, J., Hamstra, A., Arnaud, S.B., & DeLuca, H.F. (1979). Intestinal calcium absorption and serum vitamin D metabolites in normal subjects and osteoporotic patients: Effect of age and dietary calcium. *Journal of Clinical Investigation,* **64**, 729-736.

GOLDSMITH, R.S., Killian, P., Ingbar, S.H., & Bass, D.E. (1969). Effect of phosphate supplementation during immobilization of normal men. *Metabolism,* **18**, 349-368.

HALIOUA, L. (1986). High lifetime dietary calcium (Ca) intake and physical activity contribute to greater bone mineral content (BMC) and bone density (BD) in healthy premenopausal women. *Federation Proceedings,* **45**, 477.

HANSSON, T.H., Roos, B.O., & Nachemson, A. (1975). Development of osteopenia in the fourth lumbar vertebra during prolonged bed rest after operation for scoliosis. *Acta Orthopedica Scandinavica,* **46**, 621-630.

HANTMAN, D.A., Vogel, J.M., Donaldson, C.L., Friedman, R., Goldsmith, R.S., & Hulley, S.B. (1973). Attempts to prevent disuse osteoporosis by treatment with calcitonin, longitudinal compression and supplementary calcium and phosphate. *Journal of Clinical Endocrinology and Metabolism,* **36**, 845-858.

HARRISON, J.E. (1984). Neutron activation studies and the effect of exercise on osteoporosis. *Journal of Medicine,* **15**(4), 285-294.

HEANEY, R.P., Recker, R.R., & Saville, P.D. (1978). Menopausal changes in calcium balance performance. *Journal of Laboratory and Clinical Medicine,* **92**(6), 953-963.

HUDDLESTON, A.L., Rockwell, D., Kulund, D.N., & Harrison, R.B. (1980). Bone mass in lifetime tennis athletes. *Journal of the American Medical Association,* **244**, 1107-1109.

HULLEY, S.B., Vogel, J.M., Donaldson, C.L., Bayers, J.H., Friedman, R.J., & Rosen, S.N. (1971). The effect of supplemental oral phosphate on the bone mineral changes during prolonged bed rest. *Journal of Clinical Investigation,* **50**, 2506-2518.

ISSEKUTZ, B., Blizzard, J.J., Birkhead, N.C., & Rodahl, K. (1966). Effect of prolonged bed rest on urinary calcium output. *Journal of Applied Physiology,* **21**, 1013-1020.

JACOBSON, P.C., Beaver, W., Grubb, S.A., Taft, T.N., & Talmage, R.V. (1984). Bone density in women: College athletes and older athletic women. *Journal of Orthopedic Research,* **2**, 328-332.

JACOBSON, P., Beaver, W., Janeway, D., Grubb, S., Taft, T., & Talmage, R. (1984). Single and dual photon densitometry: Comparison of intercollegiate swimmers, tennis players, athletic adult women, and age-matched controls. *Transactions of the Orthopedic Research Society,* 202.

JONES, H.H., Priest, J.D., & Hayes, W.C. (1977). Humeral hypertrophy in response to exercise. *Journal of Bone and Joint Surgery,* **59A**, 204-208.

KANDERS, B., Dempster, D.W., & Lindsay, R. (1988). Interaction of calcium nutrition and physical activity on bone mass in young women. *Journal of Bone and Mineral Research,* **3**(2), 145-149.

KROLNER, B., & Toft, B. (1983). Vertebral bone loss: An unheeded side effect of therapeutic bed rest. *Clinical Science,* **64**, 537-540.

KROLNER, B., Toft, B., Nielson, S.P., & Tondevold, E. (1983). Physical exercise as prophylaxis against involutional vertebral bone loss: A controlled trial. *Clinical Science,* **64**, 541-546.

KROLNER, B., Tondevold, E., Toft, B., Berthelson, B., & Nielsen, S.P. (1982). Bone mass of the axial and the appendicular skeleton in women with Colles' fracture: Its relation to physical activity. *Clinical Physiology,* **2**, 147-157.

LANE, N.E., Block, D.A., Jones, H.H., Marshall, W.H., Wood, P.D., & Fries, J.F. (1986). Long-distance running, bone density, and osteoarthritis. *Journal of the American Medical Association,* **255**, 1147-1151.

LANYON, L.E. (1984). Functional strain as a determinant for bone remodeling. *Calcified Tissue International,* **36**, S56-S61.

LEACH, C.S., & Rambaut, P.C. (1975). Biochemical observations of long duration manned orbital spaceflight. *Journal of the American Medical Women's Association,* **30**, 153-172.

LEACH, C.S., Rambaut, P.C., & Deferranti, N. (1979). Amino aciduria in weightlessness. *Acta Astronautica,* **6**, 1323.

LINDQUIST, O., Bengtsson, C., Hansson, T., & Roos, B. (1979). Age at menopause and its relation to osteoporosis. *Maturitas,* **1**, 175-181.

LUTWAK, L., Whedon, G.D., LaChance, P.A., Reid, J.M., & Lipscomb, H.S. (1969). Mineral, electrolyte and nitrogen balance studies of the Gemini-VII fourteen-day orbital spaceflight. *Journal of Clinical Endocrinology and Metabolism,* **29**, 1140-1156.

MAINI, P.S., Lambda, R.S., & Singh, M. (1980). A study of etiological factors in osteoporosis using the femoral trabecular pattern index. In R.B. Mazess (Ed.), *Fourth International Conference on Bone Measurement* (NIH Pub. No. 80-1938, pp. 412-416). Washington, DC: U.S. Government Printing Office.

MARGULIES, J.Y., Simkin, A., Leichter, I., Bivas, A., Steinberg, R., Giladi, M., Stein, M., Kashtan, H., & Milgrom, C. (1986). Effect of intense physical activity on the bone-mineral content in the lower limbs of young adults. *Journal of Bone and Joint Surgery,* **68A**(7), 1090-1093.

MONTOYE, H.J. (1975). Relationship of osteoporosis in later life to habitual physical activity. In H.J. Montoye (Ed.), *Physical activity and health: An epidemiologic study of an entire community* (pp. 152-161). Englewood Cliffs, NJ: Prentice-Hall.

MONTOYE, H.J., McCabe, J.F., Metzner, H.L., & Garn, S.M. (1976). Physical activity and bone density. *Human Biology, 48*, 599-610.

MONTOYE, H.J., Smith, E.L., Fardon, D.F., & Howley, E.T. (1980). Bone mineral in senior tennis players. *Scandinavian Journal of Sports Science, 2*, 26-32.

NIH (1984). Consensus Development Conference on Osteoporosis. 5(3).

NILSSON, B.E., & Westlin, N.E. (1971). Bone density in athletes. *Clinical Orthopedics and Related Research, 77*, 177-182.

NORDIN, B.E.C., Wilkinson, R., Marshall, D.H., Gallagher, J.C., Williams, A., & Peacock, M. (1976). Calcium absorption in the elderly. *Calcified Tissue Research, 215*, 422-451.

OVERTON, T.R., Hangartner, T.N., Heath, R., & Ridley, J.D. (1981). Effect of physical activity on bone: Gamma ray computed tomography. In H.F. DeLuca, H.M. Frost, W.S.S. Jee, C.C. Johnston, & A.M. Parfitt (Eds.), *Osteoporosis: Recent advances in pathogenesis and treatment* (pp. 147-158). Baltimore: University Park Press.

OYSTER, N., Morton, M., & Linnell, S. (1984). Physical activity and osteoporosis in post-menopausal women. *Medicine and Science in Sports and Exercise, 16*(1), 44-50.

PARFITT, A.M. (1987). Bone remodeling and bone loss: Understanding the pathophysiology of osteoporosis. *Clinical Obstetrics and Gynecology, 30*(4), 789-811.

POCOCK, N.A., Eisman, J.A., Sambrook, P.N., Yeates, M.G., Freund, J., & Guinn, T. (1987). Muscle strength and physical fitness in the determination of bone mass (abstract). *Journal of Bone and Mineral Research, 2*(suppl. 1).

POCOCK, N.A., Eisman, J.A., Yeates, M.G., Sambrook, P.N., & Eberl, S. (1986). Physical fitness is a major determinant of femoral neck and lumbar spine bone mineral density. *Journal of Clinical Investigation, 78*, 618-621.

POGRUND, H., Bloom, R.A., & Weinberg, H. (1986). Relationship of psoas width to osteoporosis. *Acta Orthopedica Scandinavica, 57*, 208-210.

PRIEST, J.D., Jones, H.H., Tichnor, C.J.C., & Nagel, D.A. (1977). Arm and elbow changes in expert tennis players. *Minnesota Medicine, 60*, 399-404.

RAGAN, C., & Briscoe, A.M. (1964). Effect of exercise on the metabolism of ^{40}calcium and ^{47}calcium in man. *Journal of Clinical Endocrinology and Metabolism, 24*, 385-392.

RAMBAUT, P.C., Leach, C.S., & Johnson, P.C. (1975). Calcium and phosphorus changes of the Apollo 17 crewmembers. *Nutrition and Metabolism, 18*, 62-69.

RAMBAUT, P.C., Smith, M.C., Mack, P.B., & Vogel, J.M. (1975). Skeletal response. In R.S. Johnston, L.F. Dietlein, & C.A. Berry (Eds.), *Biomedical results of Apollo* (pp. 303-322). Washington, DC: NASA.

RUNDGREN, A., Aniansson, A., Ljungberg, P., & Wetterqvist, H. (1984). Effects of a training programme for elderly people on mineral content of the heel bone. *Archives of Gerontology and Geriatrics, 3*, 243-248.

SANDLER, R.B., LaPorte, R., Sashin, D., Cauley, J., Bayles, C., Slemenda, C., Petrini, A., & Schramm, M. (1984). The epidemiology of physical activity and postmenopausal bone loss: First year of a clinical trial. In C. Christianson, C.D. Arnaud, B.E.C. Nordin, A.M. Parfitt, W.A. Peck, & B.L. Riggs (Eds.), *Osteoporosis* (pp. 317-322). Glostrup, Denmark: Aalburg Striftsbogtrykkeri.

SCHNEIDER, V.S., & McDonald, J. (1984). Skeletal calcium homeostatis and countermeasures to prevent disuse osteoporosis. *Calcified Tissue International, 36*, S151-S154.

SIDNEY, K.H., Shephard, R.J., & Harrison, J.E. (1977). Endurance training and body composition of the elderly. *American Journal of Clinical Nutrition, 30*, 326-333.

SIMKIN, A., Ayalon, J., & Leichter, I. (1986). Increased trabecular bone density due to bone-loading exercises in postmenopausal osteoporotic women. *Calcified Tissue International, 40*, 59-63.

SINAKI, M., McPhee, M.C., Hodgson, S.F., Merritt, J.M., & Offord, K.P. (1986). Relationship between bone mineral density of spine and strength of back extensors in healthy postmenopausal women. *Mayo Clinic Proceedings, 61*, 116-122.

SINAKI, M., Opitz, J.L., & Wahner, H.W. (1974). Bone mineral content: Relationship to muscle strength in normal subjects. *Archives of Physical Medicine and Rehabilitation, 55*, 508-512.

SMITH, E.L., Gilligan, C., Shea, M.M., Ensign, C.P., & Smith, P.E. (in preparation). *Exercise reduces bone involution in middle-aged women.*

SMITH, E.L., Reddan, W., & Smith, P.E. (1981). Physical activity and calcium modalities for bone mineral increase in aged women. *Medicine and Science in Sports and Exercise, 13*(1), 60-64.

SMITH, M.C., Rambaut, P.C., Vogel, J.M., & Whittle, M.W. (1977). Bone mineral measurement—Experiment MO78. In R.S. Johnston & L.F. Dietlein (Eds.), *Biomedical results from Skylab* (pp. 183-190). Washington, DC: NASA Document SP-377.

STILLMAN, R.J., Lohman, T.G., Slaughter, M.H., & Massey, B.H. (1986). Physical activity and bone mineral content in women aged 30 to 85 years. *Medicine and Science in Sports and Exercise, 18*(5), 576-580.

STUPAKOV, G.P., Kazaykin, V.S., Kozlovsky, A.O., & Korolev, V.V. (1984). Evaluation of changes in human axial skeletal bone structures during long-term spaceflights. *Kosm Biol Aviakosm Med, 18*, 33.

TILTON, F.E., Degioanni, J.J.C., & Schneider, V.S. (1980). Long-term follow-up of Skylab bone demineralization. *Aviation, Space and Environmental Medicine, 51*, 1209-1213.

VOGEL, J.M. (1975). Bone mineral measurement: Skylab experiment N-078. *Acta Astronautica, 2*, 129-139.

VOGEL, J.M., & Whittle, M.W. (1976). Bone mineral changes: The second manned Skylab mission. *Aviation, Space and Environmental Medicine, 47*, 396-400.

WATSON, R.C. (1974). Bone growth and physical activity in young males. In R.B. Mazess (Ed.), *International Conference on Bone Mineral Measurements* (DHEW #NIH 75-683, pp. 380-385). Washington, DC: U.S. Government Printing Office.

WHEDON, G.D. (1984). Disuse osteoporosis: Physiological aspects. *Calcified Tissue International, 36*, S146-S150.

WHEDON, G.D., Lutwak, L., Reid, J., Rambaut, P., Whittle, M., Smith, M., & Leach, C. (1974). Mineral and nitrogen metabolic studies on Skylab orbital space flights. *Transactions of the Association of American Physicians, 87*, 95-110.

WHITE, M.K., Martin, R.B., Yeater, R.A., Butcher, R.L., & Radin, E.L. (1984). The effects of exercise on the bones of postmenopausal women. *International Orthopaedics, 7*, 209-214.

WILLIAMS, J.A., Wagner, J., Wasnich, R., & Heilbrun, L. (1984). The effect of long-distance running upon appendicular bone mineral content. *Medicine and Science in Sports and Exercise, 16*, 223-227.

YANO, K., Wasnich, R.D., Vogel, J.M., & Heilbrun, L.K. (1984). Bone mineral measurements among middle-aged and elderly Japanese residents in Hawaii. *American Journal of Epidemiology, 119*, 751-764.

ZANZI, I., Colbert, C., Batchell, R., Thompson, K., Aloia, J., & Cohn, S. (1980). Comparison of total-body calcium with radiographic and photon absorptiometry measurements of the appendicular bone mineral content. In R.B. Mazess (Ed.), *Fourth international conference on bone measurement* (NIH Pub. No. 80-1938). Washington, DC: U.S. Government Printing Office.

ZANZI, I., Ellis, K.J., Aloia, J., & Cohn, S.H. (1981). Effect of physical activity on body composition. In H.F. DeLuca, H.M. Frost, W.S.S. Jee, C.C. Johnston, & A.M. Parfitt (Eds.), *Osteoporosis: Recent advances in pathogenesis and treatment* (pp. 139-146). Baltimore: University Park Press.

Physical Activity Patterns in Older Individuals

Steven N. Blair, Patricia A. Brill, and Harold W. Kohl, III
Institute for Aerobics Research, Dallas

HEALTH BENEFITS OF PHYSICAL ACTIVITY

Several chapters in this volume deal with specific health benefits of physical activity. Herein, we briefly review some of the data on physical activity as it relates to mortality and to functional capacity.

Physical Activity and Mortality

Numerous studies over the past three decades have examined the relationship of physical activity to cardiovascular disease and all-cause mortality (Blair & Oberman, 1987). Many of these studies followed populations of middle-aged individuals and few had sufficient power to examine age-specific mortality in older individuals. In the past few years, however, more analyses have focused specifically on older cohorts. These studies are reviewed here.

Alameda County Study. A representative sample of 6,928 adult residents of Alameda County, California, has been followed since 1965 (Kaplan, Seeman, Cohen, Knudsen, & Guralnik, 1987). Numerous reports from this long-term study show all-cause mortality to be significantly and positively associated with smoking, poor sleep habits, physical inactivity, relative overweight, immoderate alcohol intake, not eating breakfast, and regular snacking, all of which are presumably adverse health behaviors or sequelae of adverse behaviors. In a recent analysis focusing specifically on older persons, Kaplan et al. (1987) show a relative risk of 1.38 for all-cause mortality in sedentary compared to physically active individuals after adjustment for other risk factors and demographic characteristics. Age-specific risk analyses for physical activity and all-cause mortality from the Alameda County Study are shown in Table 1. The relative risks are similar across the several age groups, and three of the four are significantly elevated.

Harvard Alumni Study. Paffenbarger, Hyde, Wing, and Hsieh (1986) followed 16,936 Harvard alumni for up to 16 years to measure all-cause mortality. Baseline physical activity status was assessed by questionnaire, and from these data leisure-time physical activity in kilocalories per week was estimated. All-cause mortality relative risks by specific age groups in the Harvard Alumni Study are shown in Figure 1. The most active men in the two oldest age groups (60–69 years and 70–84 years) had about 50% of the risk of dying prematurely com-

Table 1

Age-Specific All-Cause Mortality by Physical Activity Status, Men and Women, by Age Group

Age group (yrs)	Relative risk*	95% Confidence interval
38–49	1.48	1.08 - 2.02
50–59	1.27	0.97 - 1.16
60–69	1.38	1.09 - 1.75
70 +	1.37	1.09 - 1.72

Note. Adapted from "Mortality among the elderly in the Alameda County Study: Behavioral and demographic risk factors" by G.A. Kaplan, T.E. Seeman, R.D Cohen, L.D. Knudsen, & J. Guralnik, 1987, *American Journal of Public Health*, **77**, p. 309.
*Adjusted for sex, baseline health status, and behavioral risk factors.

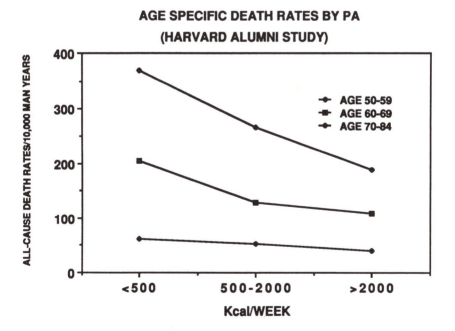

Figure 1 — Age-specific death rates from all causes in 16,936 Harvard Alumni Study over 16 years of follow-up, according to physical activity levels in kilocalories per week. Adapted from Paffenbarger et al. (1986).

pared to the least active men. The corresponding risks were about 65% in the 50–59-year age group and 80% (although not shown) in the 35–49-year age group. Thus the risk of dying prematurely in the active men was reduced in older age groups, while active men at any age were less likely to die prematurely than inactive men.

British Civil Servants. Morris, Everitt, Pollard, Chave, and Semmence (1980) recorded 475 fatal heart attacks in 17,944 middle-aged office workers over a span of 8.5 years of follow-up. Physical activity diaries completed at baseline were used to identify men who engaged in vigorous exercise (VE) in their leisure time. In this study, VE was defined as sports and recreation participation for longer than 5 minutes on a given day or a form of heavy work lasting longer than 30 minutes (e.g., gardening, lifting). The age-specific percentage of VE men and sedentary men who had fatal heart attacks during follow-up is shown in Table 2. Two important conclusions emerge from these data: First, the difference in death rates between active and sedentary men increases across the age strata; second, vigorous exercise apparently offers more protection in older men than in younger men, since the rate of fatal heart attacks in the oldest group of vigorous exercisers was lower than that of the youngest men in the no-vigorous-exercise group.

Honolulu Heart Study. In a fourth study, conducted in 1965, physical activity was assessed in 7,644 men ages 45 to 70 years (Donahue, Abbott, Reed, & Yano, 1988). Clinical coronary heart disease developed in 444 men during follow-up. In men 65 to 70 years of age, the relative risk of developing coronary heart disease was 0.41 (95% confidence limits = 0.18 to 0.95) in those who were active in 1965 compared to those who were inactive. There was a smaller reduction in risk (0.69, 95% confidence limits = 0.54 to 0.88) for active men in the 45–64 age stratum.

Mortality Summary. Thus, these four large epidemiologic studies of physical activity and mortality in groups of older men suggest an inverse relation

Table 2

Fatal Heart Attacks in Male British Civil Servants by Vigorous Exercise Status

Age-group (yrs)	Number of deaths	Reporting vigorous exercise	No vigorous exercise
40–49	138	0.8*	1.7*
50–54	129	1.3	2.9
55–65	208	1.5	5.0

Note. Adapted from "Vigorous exercise in leisure-time: Protection against coronary heart disease" by J.N. Morris, M.G. Everitt, R. Pollard, S.P.W. Chave, & A.M. Semmence, 1980, *Lancet*, II, p. 1208.
*Values are the percent of men in the category who had a fatal heart attack.

of mortality and physical activity in this age stratum. Although this may not be particularly surprising to the reader, we believe this consistency to be encouraging for at least one reason: the measurement of physical activity exposure.

Each of the studies assessed exposure to physical activity in four very different ways. A person was classified as active in the Alameda County Study if he or she reported being at least "sometimes" active in his/her leisure time. The Harvard Alumni Study classified a person's *total* energy expenditure per day in kilocalories. British civil servants were classified as vigorous exercisers if they reported sports and exercise participation over 5 minutes in duration or other forms of heavy work (e.g., gardening or jobs around the house) on a given day. Finally, the Honolulu Heart Study defined a weighted physical activity index based on a subject's usual 24-hour physical activity pattern (e.g., sleep and sedentary habits).

Obviously, there is a wide range of sensitivity in these measures and they may in fact not all be measuring the same construct of physical activity. Indeed, a recent study identified over 30 different methods to assess physical activity and its construct (LaPorte, Montoye, & Caspersen, 1985). We believe it is remarkable that despite the overall crudeness of assessment across all studies and the major differences in assessment between studies, the inverse relationship between activity and mortality is consistent, graded, and strong. Thus, with improved methods of activity assessment, the observed association will come into clear focus.

Physical Activity and Functional Capacity

Physical activity is causally associated with physical work capacity (PWC) (American College of Sports Medicine, 1986). Maintenance of PWC in the later years may have important implications for functional capability and avoidance of relative disability.

Age and PWC. PWC declines with advancing age. We studied physiologic responses to maximal treadmill testing (used as a marker of PWC) in 3,552 women ages 18 to 75 years (Blair, Lavey, Goodyear, Gibbons, & Cooper, 1984). PWC was approximately 10% lower with each successive age decade. Active women had PWC equivalent to inactive women approximately 20 years younger; that is, a 55-year-old active woman was about as fit as a sedentary 35-year-old woman. We observe similar results in middle-aged and older men. An analysis of PWC in approximately 4,500 men over 40 years of age showed a 10% decline per decade and a 20-year difference in PWC between active and sedentary men. Thus, physical activity appears to modify the decline of PWC with age.

PWC is important for functional capability as it relates to routine household, occupational, and recreational tasks. Average daily energy expenditure is probably limited to a rate of 20–30% of PWC. That is, if PWC is assessed as a $\dot{V}O_2$ max of 30 ml $\times$ kg^{-1} $\times$ min^{-1}, the average energy expenditure over the course of waking hours is limited to 6 to 9 ml $\times$ kg^{-1} $\times$ min^{-1}. Another way to view this concept is that PWC or $\dot{V}O_2$ max defines or limits a person's lifestyle from an energy expenditure perspective. Persons with high PWC simply have more energy to spend on their routine daily activities.

Limitations on daily energy expenditure do not impose problems for most individuals, especially those who are young and middle-aged. For the least fit, however, there may be adverse consequences. Kohl, Moorefield, and Blair (1987) reported an inverse association between physical fitness and prevalence of chronic fatigue in a group of low-fitness men and women. Even relatively sedentary lifestyles may stress the least fit individuals.

Low fitness may be even more of a problem for the elderly. Shephard (1979) estimates that a $\dot{V}O_2$ max of 15–16 ml $\times$ kg^{-1} $\times$ min^{-1} is necessary to maintain independent living status. According to Shephard, if a person's $\dot{V}O_2$ max falls below this standard, he or she will no longer have the capacity to handle routine self-care and household tasks, and institutionalization or home care will be required. Whether or not Shephard has selected the correct standard is somewhat irrelevant; the principle illustrated is clear. If fitness level declines too much, people become unable to take care of themselves. Additional research is needed to confirm or revise Shephard's standard, but it is a useful criterion to use until supplanted by other studies. In our data, a substantial proportion of inactive individuals reach 15–16 ml $\times$ kg^{-1} $\times$ min^{-1} by the age of 80. Few active persons are likely ever to fall below this level.

Relative Disability. Many elderly persons have various functional disabilities. The National Institute on Aging sponsored three community studies of elderly individuals. Representative community samples were surveyed in East Boston, New Haven, and rural Iowa (Coroni-Huntley, Brock, Ostfeld, Taylor, & Wallace, 1986). Participants were asked if they needed assistance with several routine activities. A summary of selected responses is given in Table 3. Most individuals over 80 years of age (men, 57%; women, 70%) need assistance with heavy housework, and many need help with climbing stairs or walking. Some, or perhaps even a majority, of the relative disability illustrated in Table 3 is due to chronic disease. Coronary heart disease, stroke, and pulmonary disease can all contribute to the inability to perform routine daily activities. We hypothesize that at least some of the relative disability is due to poor physical fitness. Low PWC and musculoskeletal fitness are probably both important in relation to disability.

Functional Capacity Summary. The data reviewed in this section suggest the importance of physical fitness as it relates to performance of daily activities and avoidance of disabilities. Much more research is needed to define the fitness standards required for independent daily function. Preventing or at least retarding the development of disability and loss of independence could have profound medical, social, and financial effects as our society ages. Suppose, for example, that it becomes possible to delay by 1 or 2 years the entrance of elderly persons into nursing homes. The benefits are obvious and could be substantial.

THE U.S. SURGEON GENERAL'S 1990 OBJECTIVES

The U.S. Surgeon General has published an extensive list of objectives for improving the nation's health (Powell, Spain, Christenson, & Mollenkamp, 1986). There are 226 discrete objectives in 15 categories. One of the categories is physical fitness and exercise. There are 11 specific objectives in this area, and 2 objectives relate to physical activity in older persons: (a) By 1990, the proportion of adults 18–65 years old participating regularly in vigorous physical activity should be greater than 60%. (b) By 1990, 50% of adults 65 years and older should be engaging in appropriate physical activity, for example regular walking, swimming, or other aerobic activity.

Table 3

Physical Function and Disability in Three Elderly White Populations

| | East Boston age groups (yrs) | | | | New Haven age groups (yrs) | | | | Rural Iowa age groups (yrs) | | | |
| | 80–84 | | > 85 | | 80–84 | | > 85 | | 80–84 | | > 85 | |
Activity	Men	Women	Men	Women	Men	Women	Men	Women	Men	Women	Men	Women
Walk across room	12*	23	22	38	8	9	10	31	10	15	17	22
Get from bed to chair	4	14	11	22	1	8	5	14	8	9	8	9
Climb stairs	15	31	29	50	12	12	10	30	12	17	16	26
Do heavy housework	57	70	74	89	31	54	53	68	43	56	68	69
Use the toilet	3	12	12	19	2	5	1	8	6	8	7	10

Note. Adapted from "Established populations for epidemiologic studies of the elderly: Resource data book." By J. Coroni-Huntley, D.B. Brock, A.M. Ostfeld, J.O. Taylor, & R.B. Wallace, 1986, National Institute on Aging, U.S. Public Health Service (NIH Publication No. 86-2443). Washington, DC: U.S. Government Printing Office.

*Values are percent of individuals needing assistance to perform the activity.

These statements are used as official evaluation standards by the U.S. Public Health Service to ascertain progress toward the 1990 objectives. Powell et al. (1986) estimate that only about 10–20% of persons in the U.S. currently meet the two objectives, and they rate the chance of achieving these objectives by 1990 as poor. It can be argued whether or not these objectives are most appropriate in terms of the public's health. Nonetheless, the objectives may serve as a useful standard against which progress can be measured.

PHYSICAL ACTIVITY PATTERNS

In order to measure progress toward national goals of physical fitness, it is necessary to accurately assess trends and patterns in physical activity. In this section we review cross-sectional and longitudinal studies on physical activity patterns in older individuals. Data from representative national samples and from specific opportunistic study groups will be used.

Cross-Sectional Surveys

Five-City Project. The Stanford University Five-City Project is a community health education program designed to prevent coronary heart disease. As part of program evaluation, four communities in northern and central California participated in a health survey in 1980. Approximately 500 households were randomly selected in each community, and 2,504 persons (65% response rate) ages 11 to 74 years were surveyed. Physical activity was assessed by a 7-day physical activity recall and by additional specific questions on moderate and vigorous physical activities (Blair et al., 1985). Moderate activity was defined as requiring 3–5 METs (work metabolic rate/rest metabolic rate), and participants were asked about their usual participation in six specific activities (including walking instead of driving for a short distance, climbing stairs instead of using the elevator, and walking during the lunch hour).

Approximately 85% of the men and women reported at least one moderate activity. The mean number of moderate activities reported varied from 1.6 to 2.0, with only slight differences between men and women and across age groups (Sallis et al., 1985). Vigorous activities ($\geq$ 6 METs) involve walking, running, or jogging at least 10 miles/week or the equivalent in other vigorous activities or sports. Only 8% of women and 25% of men reported any vigorous activities, and there was a striking decline across age groups.

Total hours per week in moderate (3–5 METs), hard (5.1–6.9 METs), and very hard ($\geq$ 7 METs) activities were ascertained by the 7-day physical activity recall (Blair et al., 1985). Results for men and women ages 35 to 74 years are shown in Table 4. There is a marked decline in all activity categories across age groups. In the 65–74-year age group, men report approximately 1 hour per day of moderate or greater activity and women report approximately 30 minutes per day.

Behavioral Risk Factor Surveys (BRFS). The Centers for Disease Control manages the BRFS in conjunction with various state health departments (White, Powell, Hogelin, Gentry, & Forman, 1987). The survey is administered by telephone interview to representative samples of adults in 28 states and the District of Columbia, with a supplemental survey covering the remaining states (except Hawaii). Through 1986 some 22,236 respondents 18 years or older were

Table 4

Hours Per Week in Moderate, Hard, and Very Hard Activity in Four California Communities

Activity level	Age group (yrs)		
	35–49	50–64	65–74
Moderate			
Men	9.7 ± 0.67*	7.9 ± 0.74	5.8 ± 1.14
Women	6.4 ± 0.52	5.9 ± 0.51	3.6 ± 0.79
Hard			
Men	4.1 ± 0.54	3.5 ± 0.60	1.6 ± 0.91
Women	1.2 ± 0.20	1.0 ± 0.19	0.3 ± 0.30
Very hard			
Men	2.0 ± 0.32	1.0 ± 0.36	0.4 ± 0.54
Women	0.1 ± 0.10	0.2 ± 0.10	0.1 ± 0.15
Number			
Men	233	191	82
Women	252	268	111

Note. Adapted from "Physical activity assessment methodology in the Five-City Project" by J.F. Sallis et al., 1985, *American Journal of Epidemiology*, **121**, p. 98.
*Values are means ± standard error.

asked about their usual type of physical activity and the hours per week they participated in each activity. Energy expenditure in kilocalories per kilogram of body weight per day was estimated from survey responses. Respondents were categorized into three groups: inactive = 0 kcal × kg^{-1} × day^{-1} in physical activity; moderately active = < 3 kcal × kg^{-1} × day^{-1}; and active ≥ 3 kcal × kg^{-1} × day^{-1}. Results, as presented in Table 5, indicate that men are more active than women, younger persons are more active than older persons, and high educational level is associated with a higher degree of physical activity.

Canada Fitness Survey. One of the most extensive surveys on a nation's physical activity pattern was done in Canada in 1981 (Stephens, Craig, & Ferris, 1986). Households ($n = 13,500$) were randomly selected for participation, and 11,800 households were contacted by the survey teams. Approximately 22,000 persons ages 10 years and older completed the survey questionnaires, which included extensive detail on type, frequency, duration, and intensity of leisure-time physical activity. These data were used to estimate energy expenditure in kcal × kg^{-1} × day^{-1}. The investigators grouped participants as sedentary (0-1.4 kcal × kg^{-1} × day^{-1}); minimally active (1.5-2.9 kcal × kg^{-1} × day^{-1}); and adequately active (≥ 3 kcal × kg^{-1} × day^{-1}). Results for men and women 40 years and older are shown in Table 6. As with the U.S. surveys, men are more active than women, but there is little difference among age groups.

National Health Interview Survey (NHIS). The NHIS is an ongoing survey of the National Center for Health Statistics, a branch of the U.S. Public

Table 5

Leisure Time Energy Expenditure by Age, Sex, and Education, BRFS

Variable	0 KKD*	0.1–2.9 KKD	≥ 3KKD
Sex			
Men	33.3 (31.1-35.4)**	39.8 (37.3-42.3)	27.0 (24.7-29.3)
Women	38.5 (36.8-40.2)	45.1 (43.2-47.0)	16.4 (14.8-18.0)
Age (yrs)			
18–34	19.1 (16.9-21.3)	52.8 (50.1-55.5)	28.2 (26.0-30.4)
35–54	37.2 (34.6-39.8)	44.8 (41.9-47.7)	18.1 (15.6-20.5)
55 +	61.2 (57.9-64.5)	23.9 (20.8-27.0)	14.9 (12.2-17.3)
Education (yrs)			
< 9	65.5 (57.4-73.6)	23.3 (16.5-30.1)	11.2 (7.4-15.0)
9–11	47.9 (43.9-51.9)	34.7 (30.3-39.1)	17.5 (14.3-20.7)
12	37.8 (35.3-40.3)	41.9 (39.0-44.8)	20.4 (18.0-22.8)
13 +	26.6 (24.2-28.8)	48.1 (45.6-50.6)	25.4 (23.2-27.6)

Note. Adapted from "The behavioral risk factor surveys: IV. The descriptive epidemiology of exercise" by C.C. White, K.E. Powell, G.C. Hogelin, E.M. Gentry, & M.R. Forman, 1987, *American Journal of Preventive Medicine*, **3**, p. 306.
*KKD = kilocalories × kg^{-1} × day^{-1}; **Values are percent in category (95% confidence limits); Values are standardized for other categories.

Table 6

Energy Expenditure in Leisure-Time Physical Activity in the Canada Fitness Survey

Age group (yrs)	Sedentary (0-1.4 KKD)*	Minimally active (1.5-2.9 KKD)	Adequately (≥ 3 KKD)
40–49			
Men	66.9**	15.9	17.2
Women	69.1	16.2	14.6
50–59			
Men	66.0	16.6	17.4
Women	68.1	16.2	16.1
60 +			
Men	59.0	17.7	23.4
Women	68.8	15.8	15.8

Note. Adapted from "Adult physical activity in Canada: Findings from the Canada Fitness Survey I" by T. Stephens, C.L. Craig, & B.F. Ferris, 1986, *Canadian Journal of Public Health*, **77**, p. 287.
*KKD = kilocalories × kg^{-1} × day^{-1}; **Values are percent of respondents in category.

Health Service. Cluster sampling procedures are followed to produce a representative sample of noninstitutionalized U.S. adults. Sample sizes vary with different cycles of NHIS reported in this section and range from 12,000 to 16,000. With these sample sizes, the percentage estimates presented here are accurate within 1–2%.

Caspersen, Christensen, and Pollard (1986) recently presented physical activity data from the NHIS conducted in 1985. Participants in NHIS are a representative national sample of the U.S. population 18 years of age and older. The survey questionnaire elicited responses on the type, frequency, and duration of recent physical activity. Caspersen et al. developed detailed scoring procedures using intensity codes for each activity to estimate the percent of individuals achieving appropriate physical activity, as specified by the 1990 objectives. This unique approach results in a somewhat more stringent criterion for activity than do most previous reports. Results of the study are shown in Table 7. Again, men are slightly more likely than women to achieve appropriate activity. The percent of participants achieving appropriate activity declines across age groups from 18 to 64 years, but there is then an increase in the 65-and-older group. The percent of individuals participating in appropriate activity is low (overall about 7.5%), suggesting a more pessimistic view of physical activity habits in the United States than is reported in other surveys.

The 1975 NHIS included several questions on exercise participation (National Center for Health Statistics, 1978). The percent distributions of responses for men and women by age groups are shown in Table 8. Women are slightly more likely to profess no regular exercise (be less active) than men. Walking is the most prevalent activity for all ages and both sexes, while most other activities are considerably more prevalent in the younger age groups. Geographic varia-

Table 7

Leisure-Time Physical Activity by Sex and Age From the NHIS

	Sedentary	Irregularly active	Regularly active, but inappropriate activity	Appropriate activity
Sex				
Men	24.8*	30.9	36.2	8.1
Women	30.2	31.3	31.5	7.0
Age (yrs)				
18–29	18.3	30.1	41.5	10.1
30–44	24.2	34.5	33.7	7.7
45–64	32.7	31.9	30.8	4.7
65 +	42.6	25.0	24.9	7.5

Note. Adapted from "Status of the 1990 physical fitness and exercise objectives—Evidence from NHIS" by C.J. Caspersen, G.M. Christenson, & R.A. Pollard, 1986, *Public Health Reports,* **101,** p. 589.
*Values are percents in each category.

Table 8

Percentage Distribution of Persons by Exercise Status and Selected Exercise Characteristics: United States, 1975

Activity	Age group (yrs) 20–24		Age group (yrs) 44–64		Age group (yrs) > 65	
	Men	Women	Men	Women	Men	Women
No regular exercise	47.0	45.2	57.6	55.2	52.0	61.1
One regular exercise or more	52.7	54.6	42.0	44.6	47.3	38.7
Bicycling	14.9	17.2	6.7	6.4	4.3	1.8
Calisthenics	17.5	17.1	10.1	11.4	5.9	6.3
Jogging	10.6	4.1	3.8	1.6	3.2	0.6*
Weight lifting	10.1	1.1	2.6	0.5*	0.5*	0.4*
Swimming	18.8	15.0	8.1	7.8	4.1	1.9
Walking	31.4	36.0	31.4	34.2	39.4	33.0
Other	6.2	7.5	5.9	7.1	8.1	6.0

Note. Adapted from "Exercise and participation in sports among persons 20 years of age and over: United States, 1975." National Center for Health Statistics, 1978. *Advance Data from Vital and Health Statistics. No. 19* (DHHS Pub. No. PHS 78-1250).
*Figure does not meet standards of reliability or precision due to small sample.

Table 9

Percentage Distribution of Persons by Exercise Status and Selected Exercise Characteristics: United States, 1975

Activity	Northeast	North Central	South	West
No regular exercise	49.4	50.1	57.8	43.6
One regular exercise or more	50.4	49.6	42.0	55.8
Bicycling	10.7	14.4	7.9	11.4
Calisthenics	14.0	13.4	10.4	18.1
Jogging	4.8	4.3	4.2	6.7
Weight lifting	3.1	3.5	3.0	4.1
Swimming	14.1	10.3	10.4	13.4
Walking	36.5	34.9	28.1	38.4
Other	7.1	5.6	6.6	8.4

Note. Adapted from "Exercise and participation in sports among persons 20 years of age and over: United States, 1975." National Center for Health Statistics, 1978. *Advance Data from Vital and Health Statistics. No. 19.* (DHHS Pub. No. PHS 78-1250).

bility in exercise participation can be seen in Table 9. These data are for the entire sample. In general, residents of the South in 1975 were the least active and those in the West were the most active.

The 1984 NHIS contained a special supplement on aging (SOA) (LaCroix, 1987). Interviews were obtained on 16,148 men and women ages 55 years and older. Participants responded to a few general questions on exercise participation. Data from these questions are presented in Tables 10–12. Approximately 25% of these older persons indicated that they participated in some form of regular exercise. In general, the prevalence of exercise was lower in the older age groups.

In response to how current activity compared to that of the previous year, more persons reported reduced current activity than increased current activity. SOA participants also were asked if they had difficulty walking and getting out of the house (Table 13). Difficulty in performing these activities tended to be more prevalent in women than in men, and was higher in older age groups.

In 1985, NHIS added a supplement on health promotion and disease prevention (Thornberry, Wilson, & Golden, 1986). Participants in this sample were asked about exercise participation in the previous 2 weeks and the length of time since they had last exercised or played sports regularly. Results of these inquiries, as presented in Table 14, indicate that walking is the most frequent activity reported in persons 30 years of age and over, and older persons report less overall participation than do younger ones.

Longitudinal Surveys

Harvard Alumni Study. Paffenbarger and colleagues (1986) have followed a cohort of Harvard College alumni since 1962. Approximately 17,000

Table 10

Percentage Distributions of Older Americans Who Report Following a Regular Routine of Exercise

Age groups (yrs)	Number	Yes	No	Not answered or unknown
Men				
55–64	2,150	26	60	14
65–74	3,083	30	60	10
75–84	1,311	26	60	14
85+	249	23	47	30
Women				
55–64	2,501	27	68	5
65–74	4,010	28	67	5
75–84	2,267	24	67	9
85+	577	15	57	28

Note. Adapted from National Health Interview Survey, Supplement on Aging, 1984 (LaCroix, 1987).

Table 11

**Percentage Distributions of Older Americans
Reporting the Number of Days Each Week They Walk 1 Mile Without Resting**

Age groups (yrs)	Number	Days per week 7	2–6	≤1	Never	Unknown
Men						
55–64	2,150	19	14	17	36	14
65–74	3,083	17	15	16	41	11
75–84	1,311	14	12	12	48	14
85+	249	8	5	8	49	30
Women						
55–64	2,501	14	16	20	45	5
65–74	4,010	11	15	15	53	6
75–84	2,267	8	9	12	62	9
85+	577	4	3	5	59	29

Note. Adapted from National Health Interview Survey, Supplement on Aging, 1984 (LaCroix, 1987).

Table 12

**Percentage Distributions of Comparison of Current Exercise Levels
to 1 Year Ago in Older Americans**

Age groups (yrs)	Number	More activity	Less activity	About the same	No answer or unknown
Men					
55–64	2,150	8	11	67	14
65–74	3,083	7	14	70	9
75–84	1,311	4	19	64	12
85+	249	5	15	51	29
Women					
55–64	2,501	10	14	72	4
65–74	4,010	8	15	72	5
75–84	2,267	7	21	63	9
85+	577	4	20	48	28

Note. Adapted from National Health Interview Survey, Supplement on Aging, 1984 (LaCroix, 1987).

Table 13

**Percentage Distributions of Older Americans Who Report Difficulty
in Walking or in Getting Outside**

Age group (yrs)	Number	Difficulty walking		Difficulty getting outside	
		Yes	No	Yes	No
Men					
55–64	2,150	9	90	3	96
65–74	3,083	13	87	5	95
75–84	1,311	18	81	8	91
85+	249	32	67	22	77
Women					
55–64	2,501	10	90	4	96
65–74	4,010	15	84	7	93
75–84	2,267	26	74	15	83
85+	577	43	55	35	62

Note. Adapted from National Health Interview Survey, Supplement on Aging, 1984 (LaCroix, 1987).

men under observation completed mail questionnaires in 1962, 1966, and 1977. In addition to health habits and other behaviors, respondents reported their participation in leisure-time physical activity. Data on sports participation in the Harvard Alumni Study are shown in Figures 2 and 3.

In these analyses, "any sport activity" includes sports with low energy expenditure, including bowling and golf. Vigorous sports are activities requiring higher energy expenditure (jogging, swimming, skiing, or court sports). These longitudinal data show an increase in sports participation across time in all birth cohorts. This group is well educated and represents the middle to upper socioeconomic strata, thus it would be unwise to generalize these findings directly to the U.S. population. Nonetheless, the data illustrate that the decline in activity across age groups seen in cross-sectional studies is not necessarily the case in a population on which there have been repeated measurements. The data are further confounded by societal changes, norms, and expectations in physical activity participation during this period (Stephens, 1987).

Aerobics Center Longitudinal Study (ACLS). The ACLS is an epidemiologic follow-up of patients examined at the Cooper Clinic in Dallas. Patients have come to the clinic for preventive medical examinations and lifestyle counseling since 1970. The clinic has administered nearly 80,000 examinations since 1970, and many patients return for multiple visits. In the cohort are 701 men and 114 women over the age of 50 who have received at least six examinations at the

Table 14

Percentage Distribution of Participation in Selected Activities in the Past 2 Weeks, and Time Since Last Regular Participation

Participation	Age groups (yrs)			
	18–29	30–44	45–64	65 +
Activity in past 2 week				
Walking for exercise	43	39	39	41
Jogging or running	24	12	4	1
Calisthenics	39	28	18	12
Biking	11	9	8	5
Swimming or water exercise	7	5	3	1
Last participation				
< 1 year	8	6	4	2
1–2 years	7	7	4	3
3–4 years	4	4	3	3
5+ years	4	25	18	17
Do not exercise regularly	34	56	69	73

Note. Adapted from National Health Interview Survey, Supplement on Health Promotion and Disease Prevention (Thornberry, Wilson, & Golden, 1986).

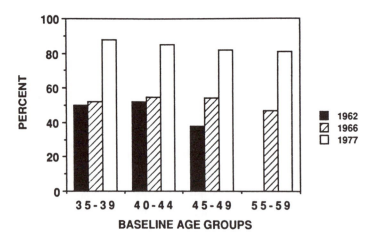

CHANGE IN ANY SPORT ACTIVITY: HARVARD ALUMNI

(Powell. Pub Health Rep 100: 118, 1985)

Figure 2 — Prevalence rates for reporting any sports activity in 1962, 1966, and 1977 in Harvard Alumni Study. Adapted from Powell and Paffenbarger (1985).

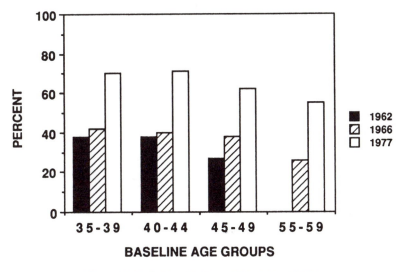

CHANGE IN VIGOROUS SPORTS: HARVARD ALUMNI

(Powell. Pub Health Rep 100: 118, 1985)

Figure 3 — Prevalence rates for reporting vigorous sports activity in 1962, 1966, and 1977 in Harvard Alumni Study. Adapted from Powell and Paffenbarger (1985).

clinic through 1987. Exercise participation was assessed by a series of questions on a medical history assessment regarding exercise participation during the month prior to the examination. Patients were classified as sedentary or active based on their responses to these questions. Cardiorespiratory fitness was assessed by a maximal treadmill test during the visit. Details on these procedures have been published previously (Blair et al., 1984).

The average interval between visits in this group was approximately 1.2 years. Data on the temporal trends in exercise habits and cardiorespiratory fitness are shown in Figures 4 and 5, respectively. The trends in these data suggest an increase in exercise participation in the cohort for both men and women. The exercise prevalence rates for women over 70 years of age are unstable due to small numbers.

The increase in reported exercise over time in the ACLS six-visit cohort is corroborated by a concomitant increase in cardiorespiratory fitness shown in Figures 4 and 5. These data must be interpreted with caution. The ACLS population is virtually all white and from middle and upper socioeconomic strata. Furthermore, the patients who return for six examinations may well be different from the overall clinic population in terms of overall health and motivation. They are likely to be more interested in their health and perhaps are more likely to adopt and maintain exercise habits. These caveats notwithstanding, our data show that older individuals can maintain, or maybe even improve, their exercise habits and cardiorespiratory fitness over a 6-year follow-up.

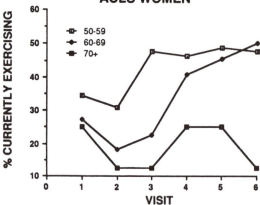

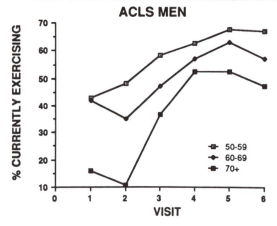

Figure 4 — Trends in self-reported exercise habits in women and men in the Aerobics Center Longitudinal Study. Number of participants: women 50–59 years = 84, 60–69 years = 22, 70+ years = 8; men 50–59 years = 568, 60–69 years = 114, 70+ years = 19.

SUMMARY

Regular physical activity is associated with good health in older individuals, and appears to provide protection against fatal coronary heart disease and to extend longevity. Numerous community and representative national surveys show less physical activity in older individuals compared to middle-aged and younger persons. Older women are particularly sedentary, according to most available data.

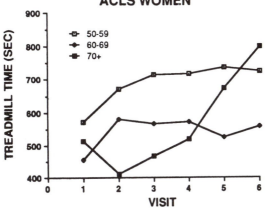

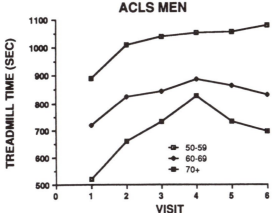

Figure 5 — Trends in maximal treadmill test time in women and men in the Aerobics Center Longitudinal Study. Number of participants: women 50–59 years = 84, 60–64 years = 22, 70+ years = 8; men 50–59 years = 568, 60–69 years = 114, 70+ years = 19.

There are very few longitudinal data on exercise and physical activity in older individuals. Existing data involve relatively select groups and thus the findings should not be generalized to the population. In these select groups, physical activity and physical fitness appear to be maintained or even increased over time in the older individuals. Much more research is needed to clarify these issues in older individuals.

REFERENCES

AMERICAN College of Sports Medicine. (1986). *Guidelines for exercise testing and prescription.* Philadelphia: Lea & Febiger.

BLAIR, S.N., Haskell, W.L., Ho, P., Paffenbarger, R.S., Jr., Vranizan, K.M., Farquhar, J.W., & Wood, P.D. (1985). Assessment of habitual physical activity by a seven-day recall in a community survey and controlled experiments. *American Journal of Epidemiology, 122,* 794-804.

BLAIR, S.N., Lavey, R.S., Goodyear, N., Gibbons, L.W., & Cooper, K.H. (1984). Physiologic responses to maximal graded exercise testing in apparently healthy white women aged 18 to 75 years. *Journal of Cardiac Rehabilitation, 4,* 459-468.

BLAIR, S.N., & Oberman, A. (1987). Epidemiologic analysis of coronary heart disease and exercise. *Cardiology Clinics, 5,* 271-283.

CASPERSEN, C.J., Christenson, G.M., & Pollard, R.A. (1986). Status of the 1990 physical fitness and exercise objectives—Evidence from NHIS 1985. *Public Health Reports, 101,* 587-592.

CORONI-HUNTLEY, J., Brock, D.B., Ostfeld, A.M., Taylor, J.O., & Wallace, R.B. (Eds.). (1986). *Established populations for epidemiologic studies of the elderly: Resource data book* (NIH Publication No. 86-2443). Washington, DC: National Institute on Aging, U.S. Public Health Service.

DONAHUE, R.P., Abbott, R.D., Reed, D.M., & Yano, K. (1988). Physical activity and coronary heart disease in middle-aged and elderly men: The Honolulu Heart Program. *American Journal of Public Health, 78,* 683-685.

KAPLAN, G.A., Seeman, T.E., Cohen, R.D., Knudsen, L.P., & Guralnik, J. (1987). Mortality among the elderly in the Alameda County Study: Behavioral and demographic risk factors. *American Journal of Public Health, 77,* 307-312.

KOHL, H.W., Moorefield, D.L., & Blair, S.N. (1987). Is cardiorespiratory fitness associated with general chronic fatigue in apparently healthy men and women? *Medicine and Science in Sports and Exercise, 19* (Suppl. 56). (abstract)

LaCROIX, A.Z. (1987). Determinants of health—Exercise and activities of daily living. In National Center for Health Statistics, R.J. Harvick, B.M. Liu, & M.G. Kovan (Eds.), *Health statistics on older persons, United States, 1986* (pp. 41-55) *Vital and Health Statistics,* Series 3, No. 25 (DHHS Publication No. PHS 87-1409). Washington, DC: U.S. Public Health Service.

LaPORTE, R.E., Montoye, H.J., & Caspersen, C.J. (1985). Measurement of physical activity in epidemiologic research: Problems and prospects. *Public Health Reports, 100,* 131-146.

MORRIS, J.N., Everitt, M.G., Pollard, R., Chave, S.P.W., & Semmence, A.M. (1980). Vigorous exercise in leisure-time: Protection against coronary heart disease. *Lancet, II,* 1207-1210.

PAFFENBARGER, R.S., Jr., Hyde, R.T., Wing, A.L., & Hsieh, C.C. (1986). Physical activity, all-cause mortality and longevity of college alumni. *New England Journal of Medicine, 314,* 605-613.

POWELL, K.E., & Paffenbarger, R.S., Jr. (1985). Workshop on epidemiologic and public health aspects of physical activity and exercise: A summary. *Public Health Reports,* **100,** 118-126.

POWELL, K.E., Spain, K.G., Christenson, G.M., & Mollenkamp, M.P. (1986). The status of the 1990 objectives for physical fitness and exercise. *Public Health Reports,* **101,** 15-21.

SALLIS, J.F., Haskell, W.L., Wood, P.D., Fortmann, S.P., Rogers, T., Blair, S.N., & Paffenbarger, R.S., Jr. (1985). Physical activity assessment methodology in the Five-City Project. *American Journal of Epidemiology,* **121,** 91-106.

SHEPHARD, R.J. (1979). Exercise and ageing. In R.S. Hutton (Ed.), *Exercise and sports sciences reviews* (pp. 1-57). Philadelphia: Franklin Institute Press.

STEPHENS, T. (1987). Secular trends in adult physical activity: Exercise boom or bust? *Research Quarterly for Exercise and Sport,* **58,** 94-105.

STEPHENS, T., Craig, C.L., & Ferris, B.F. (1986). Adult physical activity in Canada: Findings from the Canada Fitness Survey I. *Canadian Journal of Public Health,* **77,** 285-290.

THORNBERRY, O.T., Wilson, R.W., & Golden, P. (1986). Health promotion and disease prevention: Provisional data from the National Health Interview Survey: United States, January–June 1985. *Advance Data from Vital and Health Statistics,* No. 119 (DHHS Publication No. PHS 86-1250). Hyattsville, MD: Public Health Service.

WHITE, C.C., Powell, K.E., Hogelin, G.C., Gentry, E.M., & Forman, M.R. (1987). The Behavioral Risk Factor Surveys: IV. The descriptive epidemiology of exercise. *American Journal of Preventive Medicine,* **3,** 304-310.

Acknowledgments

We gratefully acknowledge the assistance of Linda Robbins and Kathyrn Henry for manuscript preparation.

Determinants of Physical Activity and Exercise for Persons 65 Years of Age or Older

Rod K. Dishman
University of Georgia

There are not enough studies, using standardized methods, to permit conclusions about the determinants of physical activity and exercise in persons 65 years of age or older. Our accumulated scientific knowledge of physical activity determinants is almost exclusively restricted to ages 18 through 64 years. Even for these ages the lack of uniformity in questions, methods, and samples renders interpretation difficult (Dishman, Sallis, & Orenstein, 1985). Because comprehensive reviews of the literature on exercise adherence are available elsewhere (Dishman, 1982, 1987, 1988a; Martin & Dubbert, 1985; Oldridge, 1982), my purpose in this paper will be to describe representative results from the few reported studies of persons 65 or older within the context of what is generally known about the determinants of physical activity and exercise. My strategy is to contrast our general knowledge with selected areas of study and application in older persons for which promising topics have not yet been fully studied or where previously unfruitful or ambiguous findings likely appear to assume more significance than has been the case for past studies of younger ages. When sufficient data in a particular area of study are available to suggest important theoretical directions or design and methodology issues for persons 65 years or older, these will be noted.

Problems inherent with assessing physical activity in the population have been reviewed extensively by others (LaPorte, Montoye, & Caspersen, 1985; Montoye & Taylor, 1984; Washburn & Montoye, 1986), so they will not be addressed here. However, physical activity assessment issues for persons 65 years or older may present unique problems due to the diversity of activity types that are appropriate for older persons and because of the unknown validity for persons 65 or older of assessment techniques widely used for ages 18 to 64 (e.g., electronic and mechanical monitors and self-reported recall).

ACTIVITY PATTERNS AND OBJECTIVES FOR THE NATION

Current population estimates (Centers for Disease Control, 1987; Stephens, 1986, 1987; Stephens, Craig, & Ferris, 1986; Stephens, Jacobs, & White, 1985; White, Powell, Hogelin, Gentry, & Forman, 1987) indicate that only 10–20% of Americans and Canadians 65 years or older are physically active at a level consistent with the U.S. 1990 Objectives for the Nation (Department of Health and Human Services, 1980). This is comparable to activity rates for the total adult population (see Figures 1 and 2). Because the 1990 objective of 50% participation by individuals 65 years and older in "appropriate" physical activity has not been met (Caspersen, Christenson, & Pollard, 1987; Powell, Spain, Christenson, & Mollenkamp, 1986), attention has been refocused on recommendations for a revised set of physical activity objectives for the year 2000 (Department of Health and Human Services, 1986, p. 37). These include the following:

1. 30% of adults 65 years of age or older will be participating in physical activity 3 or more days per week, 30 or more minutes per session, at 50% or more $\dot{V}O_2$ max (an intensity equivalent to walking about 3 miles per hour or faster).

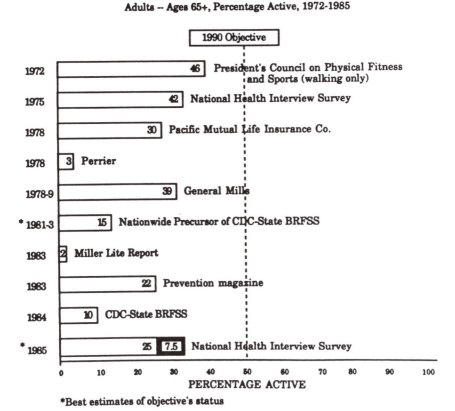

Adults -- Ages 65+, Percentage Active, 1972-1985

Figure 1 — U.S. population surveys of leisure-time physical activity for persons 65 years or older—1972-1985. Adapted from Department of Health and Human Services (1986) and Caspersen, Christenson, and Pollard (1987).

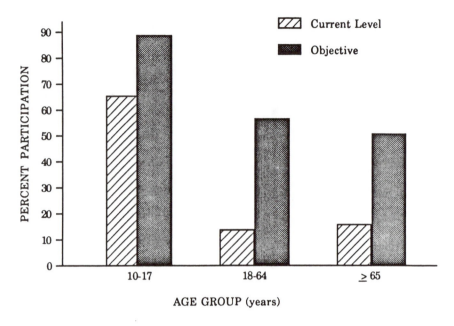

Figure 2 — **Status of the U.S. 1990 Objectives for the Nation for participation rates in leisure-time physical activity. Adapted from Powell, Spain, Christenson, and Mollenkamp (1986).**

2. 50% of adults 65 years of age or older will be participating in physical activity at least as vigorous as a sustained slow walk 3 or more days per week, 30 or more minutes per session.
3. 50% of adults 65 years of age or older will be participating 3 or more times per week for 30 minutes or more per session in activities designed to promote or maintain flexibility, ambulatory skills, arm and hand strength, or other skills of daily living.

These revised recommendations recognize that there are several major impediments to achieving their objectives. Current activity levels are low, so reaching the objectives will require increases of approximately 50–200%. There are also social and economic environments and health barriers that appear unconducive to an active lifestyle in some segments of the older population. Finally, inadequate knowledge of the determinants of physical activity makes it difficult to designate targets for effective physical activity promotions and interventions for older persons. For these reasons, recommended Physical Fitness and Exercise Objectives for the Year 2000 now include understanding the determinants of physical activity and exercise (Department of Health and Human Services, 1986). An objective for activity determinants was not included in the original 1990 objectives.

The consensus panel of the 1984 Centers for Disease Control Workshop on Epidemiologic and Public Health Aspects of Physical Activity and Exercise (Powell & Paffenbarger, 1985) recommended that several questions be addressed that are of continued importance for understanding physical activity patterns in older persons (Dishman et al., 1985). Of most relevance for this paper is the need to understand (a) how activity determinants differ according to a person's age, (b) why activity seems to diminish with advancing age and what might be done to retard this decline, (c) whether age represents a true influence on activity or represents a selection bias, and (d) who is most likely to follow and benefit from programs of vigorous exercise, from routine physical activity, and from activity modified for disabling conditions (p. 169).

WHAT IS KNOWN:
IMPLICATIONS FOR AGES 65 OR OLDER

The established determinants associated with physical activity can be organized into categories of past and present *personal attributes,* past and present *environments,* and characteristics of *physical activity* (Dishman et al., 1985). Table 1 describes these factors and their known association with leisure-time physical activity in supervised exercise programs and in the population for ages 18 to 64.

Personal Attributes

Personal attributes are predispositions that can identify people who are resistive to interventions for increasing physical activity or who are targets for interventions. Based on available evidence, blue-collar workers, low socioeconomic and low education groups, higher age groups, and individuals with high risk for CHD are relatively inactive during leisure time and are unlikely to participate in supervised exercise settings. Although the health of these groups stands to benefit greatly from increased physical activity (Larson & Bruce, 1987), these groups also appear most resistive to public health interventions of physical activity. However, because age may be a selection bias effect rather than a true determinant, and education level can be increased, these attributes may guide interventions. Other health habits and risk factors are, like physical inactivity, resistive to interventions, thus they may signal barriers to physical activity interventions rather than targets.

   The influence of personality as a determinant remains unclear but it is likely that individuals who are active and self-motivated (Dishman, Ickes, & Morgan, 1980) possess behavioral skills for setting and planning for physical activity goals, minimizing environmental barriers to implementing activity plans, self-monitoring actions, and self-reinforcement. These skills are also key components of effective self-regulatory behavior change interventions (Leventhal, Prohaska, & Hirschman, 1985). Interventions focused on psychological attributes of knowledge, attitudes, and intentions (Ajzen, 1985; Ajzen & Fishbein, 1977), health beliefs (Janz & Becker, 1984), perceptions of self-efficacy (Bandura, 1977), perceived personal control over health behaviors (Rodin, 1986), and activity outcome-expectancy values (Feather, 1982) could have a positive impact on the planning and adoption of physical activity, but they will be weak influences on maintenance if behavioral skills are not imparted that enable and reinforce behavior.

   Ages 65 or Older. The distributions of several personal attributes that are reliable correlates of physical activity and exercise for ages 18–64 are either undetermined or are different for persons age 65 or older (Brody, Brock, & Wil-

Table 1

Summary of Variables That May Determine the Probability of Leisure-Time Physical Activity and Exercise

Determinant	Changes in probability	
	Supervised program	Spontaneous program
Personal characteristics		
Past program participation	+ +	
Past extra-program activity	+	
School athletics, 1 sport	+	0
School athletics, >1 sport		+
Blue-collar occupation	– –	–
Smoking	– –	
Overweight	– –	
High risk for coronary heart disease	+ +	
Type A behavior	–	
Health, exercise knowledge	–	0
Attitudes	0	+
Enjoyment of activity	+	
Perceived health	+ +	
Mood disturbance	– –	– –
Education	+	+ +
Age	00	–
Expect personal health benefit	+	
Self-efficacy for exercise		+
Intention to adhere	0	0
Perceived physical competence	00	
Self-motivation	+ +	0
Evaluating costs and benefits	+	
Behavioral skills	+ +	
Environmental characteristics		
Spouse support	+ +	+
Perceived available time	+ +	+
Access to facilities	+ +	0
Disruptions in routine	– –	
Social reinforcement (staff, exercise partner)	+	
Family influences		+ +
Peer influence		+ +
Physical influences		+
Cost		0
Medical screening	–	
Climate	–	
Incentives	+	

(cont.)

Table 1 (cont.)

	Changes in probability	
Determinant	Supervised program	Spontaneous program
Activity characteristics		
Activity intensity	00	–
Perceived discomfort	– –	–

Note. From Dishman, Sallis, and Orenstein, 1985, ''The Determinants of Physical Activity and Exercise,'' *Public Health Reports*, **100**, 158-171.

+ + = repeatedly documented increased probability; + = weak or mixed documentation of increased probability; 00 = repeatedly documented that there is no change in probability; 0 = weak or mixed documentation of no change in probability; – = weak or mixed documentation of decreased probability; – – = repeatedly documented decreased probability. Blank spaces indicate no data.

liams, 1987). This can influence their impact as determinants or require that they be adjusted for other concomitant correlates of physical activity prior to their analyses. Distribution shifts in older persons can also result in range restrictions that reduce or eliminate individual differences and thus variability. This may require different measurement or statistical models than those used with ages 18–64. Population biases for age 65 or older include the following:

- Age—In 1982, ages 75 + were 40% of total over age 65. By the year 2000 this will be 49%. The fastest growth rate is in ages 85 or older.
- Sex—In 1982 there were 1.5 females per male for age 65 and over, and 1.06 for all ages. By the year 2000 there will be 2.34 females per male for ages 85–89.
- Race—In 1982, Caucasians were 91% of population 65 or older, and 86% of all ages.
- Social support—In 1984 some 20.2% of males and 79.8% of females 65 or older lived alone if noninstitutionalized.
- Institutional residence—In 1982 there were 1.5 million, or 5.8% of population, ages 65 or older, which translates to a current annual growth of 60,000 (Brody et al., 1987; Shephard, 1987).

Studies on Canadian men and women who are 65 years or older (Faulkner, Bailey, & Mirwald, 1987; Stones, Kozma, McNeil, & Stones, 1986) show that smoking is related to leisure-time inactivity and dropping out of exercise programs. In supervised exercise, however, the negative relationship between smoking and activity appears limited to those older persons who exercise at high intensity and frequency (Stones et al., 1986). Because of mortality and loss of interest, however, smoking is also related to dropout from studies on aging that do not include physical activity (Hirdes, Brown, Vigoda, Forbes, & Crawford, 1987). Thus, the independent effect of smoking as an influence on physical activity remains to be determined for age 65 or older. Also, because smoking and obesity are related to premature mortality in older persons, each becomes less prevalent with age, and their apparent associations with activity may thus be partly due to selection bias.

Occupation and socioeconomic status are strong correlates of physical activity in ages 18 to 64, but skewed distributions in age 65 or older occur for occupational status due to retirement, while fixed incomes among some segments of retirees may shift socioeconomic status. For these reasons, the associations for ages 65 or older of contemporary physical activity with past occupation and socioeconomic status may differ from those with current occupation and socioeconomic status. Likewise, shifts in the distribution of sex and race may present unique problems for studies of persons 65 or older. In 1982 the proportion of females in the total U.S. population was 1.06 per male. For age 65 or older there were 1.5 females per male (U.S. Bureau of the Census, 1984b). By the year 2000 it is projected there will be 2.34 females per male for ages 85 to 89. Similar findings are seen for race (U.S. Bureau of the Census, 1984a). Caucasians comprised 86% of the total U.S. population in 1982, but 91% of those age 65 or older.

Age has not been associated with adherence to supervised exercise programs among those 18 to 64, and its inverse relationship with leisure-time physical activity in the population at least partially reflects selection bias rather than a behavior influence. Prospective cohort analyses show increased activity in patients at the Cooper Clinic in Dallas (Blair, Mulder, & Kohl, 1987) and Harvard alumni ages 65–69 from 1962 to 1977 (Powell & Paffenbarger, 1985), while cross-sectional analyses of the population show that men and women ages 65 or older are more vigorously active than are those ages 50–64, even though they remain less active than those younger than 50 (Caspersen et al., 1987; Centers for Disease Control, 1987). However, for persons 65 and over, age may increasingly impose a barrier to activity. The degree to which this will reflect concomitant influences on activity due to disability, educational level, and geographic region of residence will require study (see Figure 3).

Age itself is becoming increasingly skewed toward the upper range for persons 65 years or older. In 1982, 11.6% of the U.S. population were 65 or over (Brody et al., 1987). Based on current growth rates in industrialized nations, this is expected to approach 20% in the next 50 years (Shephard, 1987). In 1985, 70% of U.S. adults survived age 65 while 30% lived to age 80 or more (Brody, 1985). By the year 2000 it is expected that persons 75 or older will comprise 50% of the total population over age 65 (U.S. Bureau of the Census, 1984a). Disability, morbidity, and mortality rates rise exponentially after age 75 (Kovar, 1977). Thus the impact of these factors on physical activity, and other activity determinants they influence, may differ for persons 65 to 74 and persons 75 years or older (see Figure 4)

Health status and physical fitness have not been reliable predictors of physical activity in ages 18–64, but the increasing prevalence of disability in persons 65 or older may reveal that limited health is a direct influence on physical activity for segments of the elderly who are disabled (Ramlow, Kriska, & LaPorte, 1987). Forty-six percent of Americans age 65 or older have at least one activity limitation (National Center for Health Statistics, 1986). Some evidence supports the

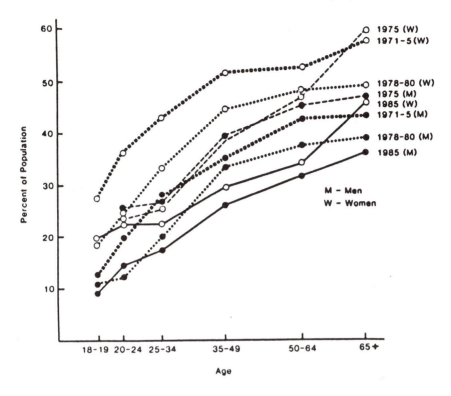

Figure 3 — **Cross-sectional estimates of the percent of U.S. adult population estimated to be sedentary across the years 1971–1985. Adapted from Stephens (1987).**

idea that physical activity is as accurate a predictor of longevity in the elderly (Kaplan, Seeman, Cohen, Knudsen, & Guralnik, 1987; Palmore, 1970) as are the risk behaviors usually associated with morbidity and mortality in middle-age (Branch & Jette, 1984; Schoenborn, 1986). Physical activity interventions thus offer the promise of increasing *active* life expectancy (Brody, 1985). Shephard (1987) has further proposed that participation by the elderly in three 1-hour exercise classes per week might reduce health care costs resulting from acute and chronic treatment, mental health costs, and extended residential care by over $600 for each senior citizen per year.

These possibilities are striking for public health, because health trends in the elderly indicate that additional years of active life expectancy are modest when compared with the more rapid increase in years lived with disabilities (Brody et al., 1987). The extent to which increased physical activity can retard disability rates or, conversely, the extent to which disability will preclude increased activity must be determined for persons 65 years or older. This distinction is particularly important for understanding the role of psychological theories as explanations of physical activity participation. Psychological dispositions to activity can be retarded or blocked by physical disability, so unavoidable barriers to activity must

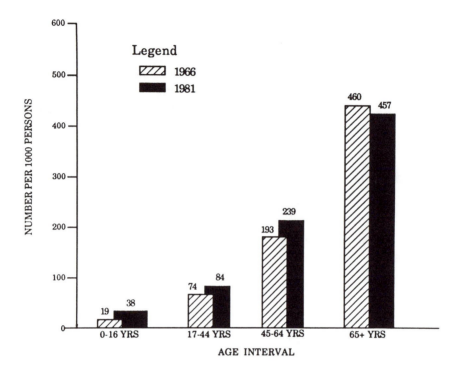

Figure 4 — Prevalence rates of activity limitation in the U.S. population for the years 1966 and 1981. Adapted from National Center for Health Statistics (1986).

be identified or controlled before the true influence of psychological determinants of activity can be assessed (Heikkinen & Kayhty, 1977).

Similarly, although there seems to be little correspondence of physical activity with other health behaviors among adults 18–64 years of age (Blair, Jacobs, & Powell, 1985; Norman, 1986), the constellations of health behaviors appear to be somewhat different for persons 65 or older (Branch & Jette, 1984; Lefebvre, Harden, Rakowski, Lasater, & Carleton, 1987; Palmore, 1970). Their enabling and reinforcing influences on physical activity could assume greater significance or different roles than for younger ages (see Figure 5). Likewise, evidence suggests that the negative impact of few years of formal education on activity in the population has decreased since the early 1970s, but this may be partly due to increased participation of persons age 65 or older (Stephens, 1987).

Past leisure-time activity is predictive of contemporary adherence to supervised exercise in middle-aged men recovering from heart attacks (Oldridge, 1982) but not in healthy men (Dishman et al., 1985), and prior leisure-time involvement in moderate activities such as walking has been predictive of supervised exercise compliance among menopausal women (Kriska et al., 1986). Trend data in the population are not available to assess the impact of past leisure-time physical activity on present leisure-time activity, but the association might be less direct

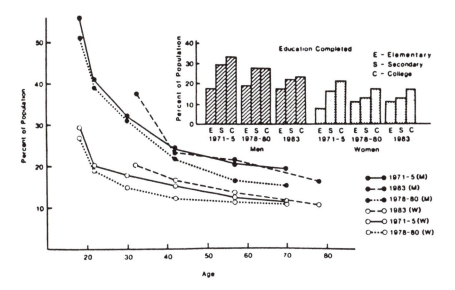

Figure 5 — Cross-sectional estimates of the percent of U.S. adults who claimed "much exercise" across the years 1971–1983. (Insert compares percentages for educational level.) Adapted from Stephens (1987).

in persons 65 or older due to occupational, economic, and medical concomitants of activity that change with age.

Although school sport participation is unrelated to contemporary leisure-time activity or supervised exercise in middle-aged Caucasian men (Dishman, 1988b), past leisure activity and sport history may assume more predictive significance in persons 65 or older. This might result from increased leisure time or decreased disability. Athletic history is not clearly linked to morbidity or mortality in males (Paffenbarger & Hyde, 1988; Stephens, Van Huss, Olson, & Montoye, 1984), but some recent evidence suggests it might be in women (Frisch et al., 1986). If so, the prevalence of past athleticism may increase in older age groups, particularly in women. Because the prevalence of heavy and overall activity in the population also increases in persons 65 or older when compared with those age 50–64, associations of these factors with physical activity in older Americans can be causal or they may reflect selection effects. This must be determined. One study of Canadian men 60–63 years of age (Stones et al., 1986) has shown higher than expected leisure physical activity in masters athletes, but the sample was too small to interpret for generalizability.

Psychological factors can account for individual differences in behavior within population segments that are demographically uniform and across different locations and times. Because psychological variables can also reflect past behavior history but can be assessed in the present, they have the potential for more precise and causal predictions of physical activity than do other personal attributes. Some psychological factors are viewed as stable traits (e.g., personality) that are relatively resistant to environmental influence, while others (e.g., attitudes, beliefs, values, expectancies, and intentions) are behavioral dispositions that are more easily changed by intervention. Prediction of a specific behavior is more accurate when psychological responses to a given situation (i.e., states) are also measured.

As for other personal attributes, too few studies of psychological determinants of physical activity are available for conclusions. However, some variables have been studied both in persons 18 to 64 years of age and in those 65 or older. For example, self-perceived mood disturbance is related to early dropout from adult fitness and cardiac rehabilitation programs among middle-aged males, while a depressive personality and somatization have also been associated with inactivity in ages 18 to 64 (Dishman et al., 1985). In general, positive mental health is associated with activity in the population, but it is unclear whether this reflects a cause, an outcome, or a selection effect. Similar results have been reported for adherence to exercise among men and women age 65 or older participating in the Philadelphia Geriatric Center (Gitlin, Lawton, Kleban, Gorman, & Windsor, 1987). Supervised attendance, compliance with an exercise intensity prescription, and maintenance of a home-based bicycling program were all predicted by low anxiety levels.

Knowledge, attitudes, intentions, outcome-expectancy values, beliefs about personal control, and efficacy in physical activity settings have essentially gone unstudied in persons 65 years or older. It has been shown, however, that elderly men and women who expect little health and fitness value from physical activity will choose to exercise at low frequency and low intensity in a supervised program (Sidney & Shephard, 1976), while those who perceive their health as poor are unlikely to join an exercise program (Shephard, 1987). Conversely, perceived gains in both fitness and health have been associated with length of supervised exercise participation among men and women 63 years of age (Stones, Kozma, & Stones, 1987). Dropping out was associated with lack of enjoyment. However, it is not known what constitutes enjoyment of exercise for persons age 65 or older, and the usefulness of emotionally based theories of motivation (e.g., Solomon, 1980) for physical activity among older persons has not been studied. Beliefs about the social appropriateness of physical activity participation may change as a function of age (Ostrow & Dzewaltowski, 1986). It is not known if these beliefs are associated with actual participation, although changes in social norms are potentially powerful determinants of physical activity for all age groups.

Perceived barriers to physical activity have also not been studied in the elderly, but they may assume increased significance due to the exponential increase in disability after age 75 (Kovar, 1977). Among persons age 18 to 64, those who perceive their health as good are more likely to enter or adhere to an exercise program, and beliefs about the ability to exercise have predicted compliance with an exercise prescription in both heart (Ewart, Stewart, Gillilan, & DeBusk, 1986) and lung (Kaplan, Atkins, & Reinsch, 1984) patients and free-living activity in a population base (Sallis et al., 1986). In older persons it will be increasingly important to distinguish perceptions of physical activity as a health-corrective behavior, whereby disease signs and symptoms can make health outcomes from exercise very salient, from perceptions of physical activity as a health-protective behavior in healthy individuals for whom health risk is more abstract and less tangible. The relative extent to which abstract thoughts and concrete feelings will prompt and reinforce physical activity may be different for persons 65 years or older than for younger persons.

Environments

Environments may be past or existing circumstances that are associated with physical activity patterns and exercise adherence; these may include perceived barriers to activity. Environments also include interventions designed to increase physical activity or exercise. It is now clear that physical activity promotions and behavior change interventions that do not address behavioral skills and environments that enable and reinforce participation cannot expect to influence determinants in a way that will maintain participation. Important components of effective interventions appear to be those that foster self-regulation of behavior (Leventhal et al., 1985), relapse preparation (Marlatt & Gordon, 1985), and tangible reinforcement of activity. Traditional health promotion and education, including medical and fitness screening or health risk appraisal (Godin & Shephard, 1983), cannot by themselves motivate participation because they focus on abstract health incentives for activity that have high potential for prompting the adoption of a health behavior but a relatively low potential for reinforcing maintenance or adherence.

Enabling environments can prompt and permit physical activity; but environments that support and tangibly reinforce behavior change, while removing barriers, are needed for maintaining a physical activity pattern (Martin & Dubbert, 1985). Normative social prompts and social support for physical activity participation are unlikely to be strong enough to maintain physical activity when concrete rewarding perceptions do not accompany physical activity.

Ages 65 or Older. Some environmental characteristics are not conducive to change but must be considered potential barriers to interventions. These characteristics may assume added significance for persons 65 or older or may create methodologic problems for interpretation. For example, the comparatively low physical activity rates found in the southern and eastern regions of the U.S. (Stephens et al., 1985) may reflect a greater proportion of older residents, low education level, or low socioeconomic level. There is no evidence that the financial cost of physical activity is a barrier to participation among ages 18 to 64 (Dishman et al., 1985; Oldridge, 1982), but cost could assume significance for certain individuals age 65 years or older due to income shifts with retirement. Similarly, spousal and social support are robust influences on supervised exercise and physical activity in the 18- to 64-year-old population, but the social environment can change dramatically for some persons in their later years (see Figure 6). In 1984, for example, 20.2% of males and 79.8% of females 65 or older who were not institutionalized lived alone (Brody et al., 1987).

Access to facilities is a necessary but insufficient facilitator of recreational physical activity. Both perceived and actual convenience of the exercise setting are reliable predictors of participation in supervised exercise programs among those age 18 to 64 (Dishman et al., 1985), yet in the U.S. population the already active are twice as likely as the inactive to state that increased access to facilities

Number of residents per 1000 population

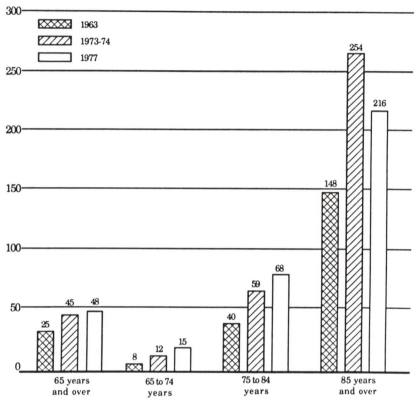

Figure 6 — Use of nursing homes by the elderly in the U.S. across age groups for the years 1963, 1973–1974, and 1977. Adapted from Brody, Brock, and Williams (1987).

would increase their activity levels (The Perrier Study, 1979). However, the elderly perceive facilities to be an important influence on activity participation (Shephard, 1987), and home-based exercise can facilitate participation for some people. Facility access may assume greater significance for those 65 or older, particularly those who are disabled or institutionalized (see Figure 7). In 1982, 1.5 million, or 5.8%, of Americans age 65 or older lived in an institution, and the current growth rate is 60,000 additional persons per year (Brody et al., 1987).

It will also be important to determine if perceptions or beliefs about available leisure time are related to physical activity among persons who are 65 or older. For ages 18 to 64, lack of time is the most prevalent reason stated for inactivity (Dishman et al., 1985), yet the inactive and active apparently have the same actual hours of weekly leisure time (The Perrier Study, 1979). Increased leisure time may partly explain why Americans and Canadians 65 years or older participate at a higher rate in leisure-time physical activity than do persons age 50 to 64.

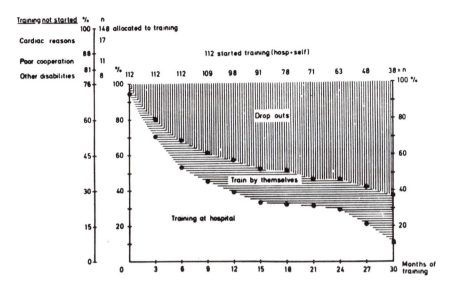

Figure 7 — Exercise adherence rates in the Goteborg, Sweden, Clinical Exercise Trial. From "Exercise tolerance and physical training of non-selected patients after myocardial infarction" by H.M. Sanne, D. Elmfeldt, G. Grimby, C. Rydin, and L. Wilhelmsen, 1973, *Acta Medica Scandinavica,* 551 (Suppl.), p. 60.

Interventions to increase physical activity among persons 65 or older have received little study, yet a supervised exercise intervention can increase peak VO_2, oxygen pulse, and high intensity (≥ 5 METS) leisure-time physical activity among men 1 year after retirement (Cunningham, Rechnitzer, Howard, & Donner, 1987). Cognitive behavior modification techniques that have been associated with increased activity in ages 18 to 64 (Knapp, 1988) should be effective for adults 65 or older, but their effectiveness has not been tested for older persons. Two studies with institutionalized geriatric samples, however, have shown that acute and chronic increases in stationary bicycle exercise are associated with token reinforcement (Libb & Clements, 1969) and with implementation of goal setting, goal posting with feedback, and token reinforcement contingent on goal attainment (Perkins, Rapp, Carlson, & Wallace, 1986). However, the increase in physical activity that accompanies behavioral interventions is typically lost within 3 months after the intervention is removed (see Figure 8).

The effective promotion of physical activity by physicians is a potentially strong determinant of physical activity for persons age 65 or older due to increased physician contact with the aging, but activity interventions in the physician's office remain poorly explained for all ages (Dishman, in press; Iverson, Fielding, Crow, & Christenson, 1985). It is recommended for the year 2000 that 65% or more of primary medical care providers inquire about the frequency, duration, type, and intensity of most new patients' exercise habits (Department of Health and Human Services, 1986). Medical office interventions deserve particular attention for older persons because, to them, a doctor's advice appears to be a more prevalent perceived reason for physical activity (Canada Fitness Survey, 1983).

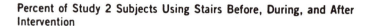

Percent of Study 2 Subjects Using Stairs Before, During, and After
Intervention

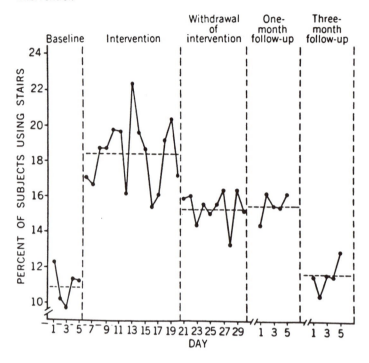

Figure 8 — Effectiveness of a public health intervention for increasing stair use at a commuter train station in Philadelphia (n = 24, 603). From "Evaluation and modification of exercise patterns in the natural environment" by K.D. Brownell, A.J. Stunkard, and J.M. Albaum, 1980, American Journal of Psychiatry, 137, p. 1542.

    Knowledge of health and exercise was associated with regular activity of moderate intensity (e.g., routine walking) for both men and women in a population-based study, but this did not predict participation in vigorous exercise (Sallis et al., 1986). Inactive members of minority and low socioeconomic groups are relatively uninformed about the health benefits of exercise and its appropriate forms or amounts (Atkins et al., 1987), but in the U.S. population only about 5% of both the currently inactive and the active believe more information on fitness benefits likely would increase their participation (The Perrier Study, 1979). Paradoxically, however, only 5% of the U.S. population can accurately identify the optimal intensity, duration, and frequency of physical activity for cardiopulmonary fitness (Caspersen et al., 1987). Although roughly 70% of Americans can identify appropriate frequency and duration for fitness, many overestimate or underestimate optimal intensity and activity types (Caspersen et al., 1987). Misconceptions among the elderly about appropriate activity types and intensity could be a particularly strong barrier to participation, due to inaccurate self-appraisals of activity level or ability to be active or to increased risk of injury.

It will thus be important to determine if these findings on knowledge from the general population hold for persons 65 or older. Until this is determined, however, it appears that education campaigns directed at persons age 65 or older may more effectively increase physical activity if they dispel misinformation that might impede activity for some groups. It is noteworthy that in 1972, even though older persons were less active, they were much more likely to believe they were getting enough exercise than were persons younger than 60 (Clarke, 1973); paradoxically, less active adults were more apt to view their activity level as adequate than were active persons. It is not known whether this finding holds today. However, the recommended Objectives for the Nation by the Year 2000 (Department of Health and Human Services, 1986) call for 80% of persons age 10 and older to know that regular physical activity reduces heart disease, obesity, depression, and anxiety as well as to know the variety, frequency, and duration of exercise that promotes cardiorespiratory fitness. These objectives may be especially relevant for public health promotions of activity in the elderly because of limited access to formal education in persons 65 or older.

Knowledge about effective goal setting will also need to be augmented by behavioral skills that are reinforced by successful experience or peer models who demonstrate the skills and desirable outcomes. Even so, knowledge of and belief in the health benefits of physical activity may motivate initial involvement, but feelings of enjoyment and well-being may be stronger motives for continued participation in gerontology exercise programs (Stones et al., 1986). The role of self-regulatory attributes and skills (Leventhal et al., 1985) in the physical activity patterns of persons 65 or older also is not known, although one study has shown self-motivation (Dishman et al., 1980) to be unrelated to activity in a geriatric sample (Gitlin et al., 1987).

Physical Activity

Physical activity types and amounts appropriate for health and for enabling and reinforcing participation must be determined for various population segments. Moderate physical activity, compared to fitness activities, is associated with a higher rate of adoption and maintenance of physical activity patterns in a population base, and this is particularly true for women (Sallis et al., 1986). In supervised exercise programs in which the intensity of activity is individualized according to fitness level, adherence appears weakly related to activity intensity or duration in the absence of injury (Pollock, 1988).

Ages 65 or Older. Physical activity objectives may vary widely for persons 65 or older. This is largely due to increased disability and activity limitations among persons 65 or older and the possibility that physical activity, more so than physical fitness, is a strong independent predictor of longevity in the elderly. Relatively low-intensity exercise (approximating 40% of $\dot{V}O_2$ max) can increase cardiorespiratory fitness in the elderly. However, added emphasis on non-weight-bearing activity, flexibility, and hand and arm strength may be more important as public health goals for physical activity and fitness among persons age 65 or older when compared with goals for ages 18–64 because of increasing disability and activity limitations after age 75 (see Table 2).

Perceived choice over activity type has been associated with increased participation in young adults (Thompson & Wankel, 1980), so increased emphasis

Table 2

A Physical Activity Plan for Improving Health and Fitness for Older Adults Over the Age of 65 Years

Major health–fitness goals	Physical activity plan[1]
Maintain general functional capacity Retain musculoskeletal integrity Enhance psychological status Prevent and treat CHD[2] and Type II diabetes	T Emphasis on moving about, flexibility, and some resistive exercise I Moderate intensity (overload with slow progression) D Based on capacity of individual, up to 60 minutes per day in multiple sessions F Every day G Lower level activities (for example, walking) every day

Note. From W.L. Haskell, H.J. Montoye, and D. Orenstein, 1985, "Physical Activity and Exercise to Achieve Health-Related Physical Fitness Components," *Public Health Reports*, **100**, p. 206.
[1]T = type of exercise; I = intensity; D = duration or amount; F = frequency of exercise session.
[2]Coronary heart disease.

on the diversity of types and amounts of physical activity for ages 65 or older (Department of Health and Human Services, 1986) may reveal parameters of physical activity to be particularly important predictors of participation for older ages.

The influence of perceived exertion on activity participation among persons 65 or older has not been studied (Dishman et al., 1985), but perceived exertion may interact with intensity prescriptions and with participants' beliefs about their personal efficacy for physical activity to influence participation. Because perceived exertion in adults 65 or older appears related to percent peak $\dot{V}O_2$ in a way comparable to that of younger persons (Sidney & Shephard, 1977), perceived exertion holds particular promise as a behaviorally based adjunct to metabolically based intensity prescriptions among persons 65 or older (see Figure 9). Alternative prescriptions related to perceived exertion or preferred exertion levels may be especially useful when disabling or activity-limiting conditions contraindicate, or delimit, the appropriateness of traditional fitness-based prescriptions that exclusively use objective measures of work load, work rate, or physiological responses to physical activity.

SUMMARY

Understanding the determinants of physical activity and exercise for persons 65 or older will be a timely and important public health objective for the coming decade and beyond. Too little is now known for conclusions, so I have attempted

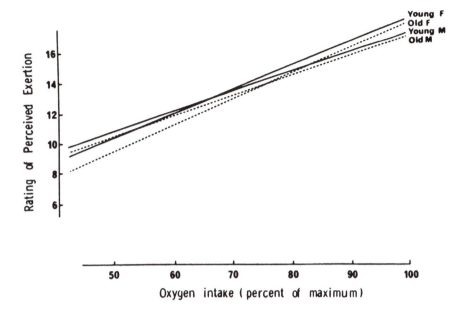

Figure 9 — Perceived exertion is comparable for elderly and young individuals when viewed as a function of relative oxygen consumption (%$\dot{V}O_2$ peak). Adapted from Sidney and Shephard (1977).

to describe representative findings for persons age 65 or older within the theoretical and empirical frameworks that characterize our knowledge of physical activity and exercise determinants for ages 18 to 64. It will be important in future studies to recognize changes in personal attributes, environments, and physical activity abilities and objectives that appear to distinguish persons 65 years or older from younger adults. Precise and valid measures of physical activity and determinants must also be developed for use in supervised and population studies with older persons. Uniform methods are needed to allow comparisons between studies for which current methods vary widely.

Several factors previously found to be weakly associated with activity patterns in younger ages may assume clearer significance in persons 65 or older. Personal attributes including disability and activity limitations, knowledge about physical activity, beliefs about exercise outcomes and outcome-expectancy values, feelings of physical control or self-efficacy in exercise settings, and environmental characteristics of facility or program access and social support may prove more important than they have for younger ages. Physical activity promotions by physicians, community agencies, and geriatric institutions may assume increasingly important roles if population trends for increased longevity with disability continue as expected. Based on established efficacy in persons 18 to 64 years of age, behavior modification interventions employing stimulus- and reinforcement-control techniques and self-regulatory skills should provide useful adjuncts to activity promotions. Their most effective applications to the elderly remain to be demonstrated for exercise and physical activity.

The expanding objectives for physical activity and exercise, as they relate to public health goals for those 65 or older, will place greater emphasis on lower intensity and more diversified types of activity than has been the case for ages 18 to 64. Thus, many of the interactions between the determinants of physical activity and exercise among persons age 65 or older may be different from those for persons 18 to 64 years of age. These differences will place new research demands on design, analysis, and physical activity measurement. Of great significance and promise, however, is the observation that for most persons 65 years or older, increasing age is not a *cause* of physical inactivity; with due consideration of personal attributes, environments, and physical activity abilities and goals unique to persons 65 years or older, our national participation goals for the year 2000 feasibly could be met.

REFERENCES

AJZEN, I. (1985). From intentions to actions. A theory of planned behavior. In J. Kuhl & J. Beckman (Eds.), *Action-control: From cognition to behavior* (pp. 11-39). Heidelberg: Springer.

AJZEN, I., & Fishbein, M. (1977). Attitude–behavior relations: A theoretical analysis and review of empirical research. *Psychological Bulletin,* **84**, 888-918.

ATKINS, C.J., Patterson, T.L., Roppe, B.E., Kaplan, R.M., Sallis J.F., & Nadar, P.R. (1987). Recruitment issues, health habits, and the decision to participate in a health promotion program. *American Journal of Preventive Medicine, 3*, 87-94.

BANDURA, A. (1977). Self-efficacy: Toward a unifying theory of behavioral change. *Psychological Review,* **84**, 191-215.

BLAIR, S.N., Jacobs, D.R., Jr., & Powell, K.E. (1985). Relationships between exercise or physical activity and other health behaviors. *Public Health Reports,* **100**, 172-180.

BLAIR, S.N., Mulder, R.T., & Kohl, H.W. (1987). Reaction to ''Secular trends in adult physical activity: Exercise boom or bust?'' *Research Quarterly for Exercise and Sport,* **58**, 106-110.

BRANCH, L.G., & Jette, A.M. (1984). Personal health practices and mortality among the elderly. *American Journal of Public Health,* **74**, 1126-1129.

BRODY, J.A. (1985). Prospects for an aging population. *Nature,* **315**, 463-466.

BRODY, J.A., Brock, D.B., & Williams, T.F. (1987). Trends in the health of the elderly population. *Annual Review of Public Health, 8*, 211-234.

CANADA Fitness Survey. (1983). *Fitness and lifestyle in Canada.* Ottawa: Fitness Canada.

CASPERSEN, C.J., Christenson, G.M., & Pollard, R.A. (1987). Status of the 1990 physical fitness and exercise objectives—Evidence from NHIS 1985. *Public Health Reports,* **101**, 587-592.

CENTERS for Disease Control. (1987). Sex-, age-, and region-specific prevalance for sedentary lifestyle in selected states in 1985—The Behavioral Risk Factor Surveillance System. *Morbidity and Mortality Weekly Reports, 36*, 195-198, 203-204.

CLARKE, H.H. (Ed.) (1973, May). National adult physical fitness survey. *President's Council on Physical Fitness and Sports Newsletter*, Special Edition, Washington, DC: U.S. Government Printing Office.

CUNNINGHAM, D.A., Rechnitzer, P.A., Howard, J.H., & Donner, A.P. (1987). Exercise training of men at retirement: A clinical trial. *Journal of Gerontology*, **42**, 17-23.

DEPARTMENT of Health and Human Services. (1980, Fall). *Promoting health/preventing disease: Objectives for the nation*. Washington, DC: U.S. Government Printing Office.

DEPARTMENT of Health and Human Service. (1986). *Midcourse review, 1990 physical fitness and exercise objectives*. President's Council on Physical Fitness and Sports and Behavioral Epidemiology Branch, Center for Health Promotion, Centers for Disease Control. Washington, DC: U.S. Government Printing Office.

DISHMAN, R.K. (1982). Compliance/adherence in health-related exercise. *Health Psychology*, **1**, 237-267.

DISHMAN, R.K. (1987). Exercise adherence and habitual physical activity. In W.P. Morgan & S.N. Goldston (Eds.) *Exercise and mental health* (pp. 59-83). Washington, DC: Hemisphere.

DISHMAN, R.K. (Ed.) (1988a). *Exercise adherence: Its impact on public health*. Champaign, IL: Human Kinetics.

DISHMAN, R.K. (1988b). Supervised and free-living physical activity: No differences in former athletes and nonathletes. *American Journal of Preventive Medicine*, **4**, 153-160.

DISHMAN, R.K., Ickes, W., & Morgan, W.P. (1980). Self-motivation and adherence to habitual physical activity. *Journal of Applied Social Psychology*, **10**, 115-132.

DISHMAN, R.K., Sallis, J.F., & Orenstein, D. (1985). The determinants of physical activity and exercise. *Public Health Reports*, **100**, 158-171.

DISHMAN, R.K. (in press). Promoting physical activity in medical care. In J. Torg, P. Welsh, & R. Shephard (Eds.), *Current therapy in sports medicine*. Philadelphia: Brian Decker Publ.

EWART, C.K., Stewart, J.K., Gillilan, R.E., & DeBusk, A. (1986). Usefulness of self-efficacy in predicting overexertion during programmed exercise in coronary artery disease. *American Journal of Cardiology*, **57**, 557-561.

FAULKNER, R.A., Bailey, D.A., & Mirwald, R.L. (1987). The relationship of physical activity to smoking characteristics in Canadian men and women. *Canadian Journal of Public Health*, **78**, 155-160.

FEATHER, N.T. (1982). *Expectations and actions: Expectancy value models in psychology*. Hillsdale, NJ: Erlbaum.

FRISCH, R.E., Wyshak, G., Albright, N.L., Albright, T.E., Schiff, I., Witschi, J., & Marguglio, M. (1986). Lower lifetime occurrence of breast cancer and cancers of the reproductive system among former college athletes. *American Journal of Clinical Nutrition*, **44**, 328-335.

GITLIN, L.N., Lawton, M.P., Kleban, M.H., Gorman, K.M., & Windsor, L.A. (1987, November 21). *Predictors of compliance to exercise: A model for healthy elderly*. Paper presented at the annual meeting of the Gerontological Society of America, Washington, DC.

GODIN, G., & Shephard, R.J. (1983). Physical fitness promotion programmes: Effectiveness in modifying exercise behavior. *Canadian Journal of Applied Sport Science*, **8**, 104-113.

HEIKKINEN, E., & Kayhty, B. (1977). Gerontological aspects of physical activity: Motivation for older people in physical training. In R. Harris & L.J. Frankel (Eds.), *Guide to fitness after 50*. New York: Plenum Press.

HIRDES, J.P., Brown, K.S., Vigoda, D.S., Forbes, W.F., & Crawford, L. (1987). Health effects of cigarette smoking: Data from the Ontario Longitudinal Study on Aging. *Canadian Journal of Public Health, 78*, 13-17.

IVERSON, D.C., Fielding, J.E., Crow, R.S., & Christenson, G.M. (1985). The promotion of physical activity in the U.S. population: The status of programs in medical, worksite, community, and school settings. *Public Health Reports, 100*, 212-224.

JANZ, N.K., & Becker, M.H. (1984). The health belief model: A decade later. *Health Education Quarterly, 11*, 1-47.

KAPLAN, G.A., Seeman, T.E., Cohen, R.D., Knudsen, L.P., & Guralnik, J. (1987). Mortality among the elderly in the Alameda County Study: Behavioral and demographic risk factors. *American Journal of Public Health, 77*, 307-312.

KAPLAN, R.M., Atkins, C.J., & Reinsch, S. (1984). Specific efficacy expectations mediate exercise compliance in patients with COPD. *Health Psychology, 3*, 223-242.

KNAPP, D.N. (1988). Behavioral management techniques and exercise promotion. In R.K. Dishman (Ed.), *Exercise adherence: Its impact on public health* (pp. 203-236). Champaign, IL: Human Kinetics.

KOVAR, M.G. (1977). Elderly people: The population 65 years and over. In *Health, United States, 1976–1977* (Publication No. HRA 77-1232). Hyattsville, MD: Department of Health, Education, and Welfare.

KRISKA, A.M., Bayles, C., Cauley, J.A., LaPorte, R.E., Sandler, R.B., & Pambianco, G. (1986). A randomized exercise trial in older women: Increased activity over two years and the factors associated with compliance. *Medicine and Science in Sports and Exercise, 8*, 557-562.

LaPORTE, R.E., Montoye, H.J., & Caspersen, C.J. (1985). Assessment of physical activity in epidemiologic research: Problems and prospects. *Public Health Reports, 100*, 131-146.

LARSON, E.B., & Bruce, R.A. (1987). Health benefits of exercise in an aging society. *Archives of Internal Medicine, 147*, 353-356.

LEFEBVRE, R.C., Harden, E.A., Rakowski, W., Lasater, T.M., & Carleton, R.A. (1987). Characteristics of participants in community health promotion programs: Four year results. *American Journal of Public Health, 77*, 1342-1344.

LEVENTHAL, H., Prohaska, T.R., & Hirschman, R.S. (1985). Preventive health behavior across the life-span. In J.C. Rosen & L.J. Solomon (Eds.), *Preventing health risk behaviors and promoting coping with illness*. Hanover, NH: University Press of New England.

LIBB, J.W., & Clements, C.B. (1969). Token reinforcement in an exercise program for hospitalized geriatric patients. *Perceptual and Motor Skills, 28*, 957-958.

MARLATT, G.A., & Gordon, J.R. (Eds.). (1985). *Relapse prevention: Maintenance strategies in the treatment of addictive behaviors*. New York: Guilford Press.

MARTIN, J.E., & Dubbert, P.M. (1985). Adherence to exercise. *Exercise and Sport Sciences Reviews,* **13**, 137-167.

MONTOYE, H.J., & Taylor, H.L. (1984). Measurement of physical activity in population studies: A review. *Human Biology,* **56**, 195-216.

NATIONAL Center for Health Statistics. (1986). *Vital and Health Statistics: National Health Interview Survey,* Series 10. Washington, DC: U.S. Government Printing Office.

NORMAN, R.M.G. (1986). *The nature and correlates of health behavior.* Health Promotion Studies Series No. 2. Ottawa: Health and Welfare Canada.

OLDRIDGE, N.G. (1982). Compliance and exercise in primary and secondary prevention of coronary heart disease: A review. *Preventive Medicine,* **11**, 56-70.

OSTROW, A.C., & Dzewaltowski, D.A. (1986). Older adults' perceptions of physical activity participation based on age-role and sex-role appropriateness. *Research Quarterly for Exercise and Sport,* **57**, 167-169.

PAFFENBARGER, R.S., Jr., & Hyde, R.T. (1988). Exercise adherence, coronary heart disease, and longevity. In R.K. Dishman (Ed.), *Exercise adherence: Its impact on public health* (pp. 41-73). Champaign, IL: Human Kinetics.

PALMORE, E. (1970). Health practices and illness among the aged. *The Gerontologist,* **1**, 313-316.

PERKINS, K.A., Rapp, S.R., Carlson, C.R., & Wallace, C.E. (1986). A behavioral intervention to increase exercise among nursing home residents. *The Gerontologist,* **26**, 479-481.

PERRIER Study, The. (1979). *Fitness in America.* New York: Perrier–Great Waters of France, Inc.

POLLOCK, M.L. (1988). Exercise prescription for fitness and adherence. In R.K. Dishman (Ed.), *Exercise adherence: Its impact on public health* (pp. 259-278), Champaign, IL: Human Kinetics.

POWELL, K.E., & Paffenbarger, R.S. (1985). Workshop on epidemiologic and public health aspects of physical activity and exercise. *Public Health Reports,* **100**, 118-126.

POWELL, K.E., Spain, K.G., Christenson, G.M., & Mollenkamp, M.P. (1986). The status of the 1990 objectives for physical fitness and exercise. *Public Health Reports,* **101**, 15-21.

RAMLOW, J., Kriska, A., & Laporte, R.A. (1987). Physical activity in the population: The epidemiologic spectrum. *Research Quarterly for Exercise and Sport,* **58**, 111-114.

RODIN, J. (1986). Aging and health: Effects of the sense of control. *Science,* **233**, 1271-1276.

SALLIS, J.F., Haskell, W.L., Fortmann, S.P., Vranizan, K.M., Taylor, C.B., & Solomon, D.S. (1986). Predictors of adoption and maintenance of physical activity in a community sample. *Preventive Medicine,* **15**, 331-341.

SCHOENBORN, C.A. (1986). Health habits of U.S. adults, 1985: The "Alameda 7" revisited. *Public Health Reports,* **101**, 571-580.

SHEPHARD, R.J. (1987). *Physical activity and aging* (2nd ed.). London: Croom Helm.

SIDNEY, K.H., & Shephard, R.J. (1976). Attitude toward health and physical activity in the elderly: Effects of a physical training program. *Medicine and Science in Sports,* **8**, 246-252.

SIDNEY, K.H., & Shephard, R.J. (1977). Perception of exertion in the elderly: Effects of aging, mode of exercise, and physical training. *Perceptual and Motor Skills,* **44**, 999-1010.

SOLOMON, R.L. (1980). The opponent process theory of acquired motivation. *American Psychologist,* **35**, 691-712.

STEPHENS, K.E., Van Huss, W.D., Olson, H.W., & Montoye, H.J. (1984). The longevity, morbidity, and physical fitness of former athletes—an update. *American Academy of Physical Education Papers* (Vol. 17, pp. 101-119). Champaign, IL: Human Kinetics.

STEPHENS, T. (1986). Health practices and health status: Evidence from the Canada Health Survey. *American Journal of Preventive Medicine,* **2**, 209-215.

STEPHENS, T. (1987). Secular trends in adult physical activity: Exercise boom or bust? *Research Quarterly for Exercise and Sport,* **58**, 94-105.

STEPHENS, T., Craig, C.L., & Ferris, B.F. (1986). Adult physical activity in Canada: Findings from the Canada Fitness Survey I. *Canadian Journal of Public Health,* **77**, 285-290.

STEPHENS, T., Jacobs, D.R., Jr., & White, C.C. (1985). A descriptive epidemiology of leisure-time physical activity. *Public Health Reports,* **100**, 147-158.

STONES, M.J., Kozma, A., McNeil, A.K., & Stones, L. (1986). Smoking behavior and participation in organized exercise. *Canadian Journal of Public Health,* **77**, 153-154.

STONES, M.J., Kozma, A., & Stones, L. (1987). Fitness and health evaluations by older exercisers. *Canadian Journal of Public Health,* **78**, 18-20.

THOMPSON, C.E., & Wankel, L.M. (1980). The effects of perceived choice upon frequency of exercise behavior. *Journal of Applied Social Psychology,* **10**, 436-443.

U.S. BUREAU of the Census. (1984a). Projections of the population of the United States, by age, sex, and race: 1983 to 2080. *Current Population Reports* (Series P-25, No. 952). Washington, DC: U.S. Government Printing Office.

U.S. BUREAU of the Census. (1984b). Demographic and socioeconomic aspects of aging in the United States. *Current Population Reports* (Series P-23, No. 138). Washington, DC: U.S. Government Printing Office.

WASHBURN, R.A., & Montoye, H.J. (1986). The assessment of physical activity by questionnaire. *American Journal of Epidemiology,* **123**, 563-576.

WHITE, C.C., Powell, K.E., Hogelin, G.C., Gentry, E.M., & Forman, M.R. (1987). The behavioral risk factor surveys: IV. The descriptive epidemiology of exercise. *American Journal of Preventive Medicine,* **3**, 304-310.

Exercise Prescriptions for the Elderly

Michael L. Pollock
University of Florida

Exercise prescription for the elderly, as for the younger person, depends on their needs, goals, physical and health status, available time, equipment, and facilities (Larson & Bruce, 1987; Pollock & Wilmore, in press; Wheat, 1987). A clear understanding of the participants' needs and goals is necessary to prescribe exercise safely and adequately. The fact that the elderly vary greatly in health and fitness status makes the art of prescribing exercise more challenging. This paper will discuss guidelines for exercise prescription for healthy, ambulatory elderly participants.

Most elderly persons can benefit from a properly designed exercise program (Badenhop, Cleary, Schaal, Fox, & Bartels, 1983; Barry et al., 1966; deVries, 1970; Miyashita, Haga, & Mitzuta, 1978; Pollock et al., 1976; Seals, Hagberg, Hurley, Ehsani, & Holloszy, 1984; Sidney, Shephard, & Harrison, 1977; Smith & Serfass, 1981). Whether one is ambulatory or bedridden, it is important to stay as functionally active as possible. Even low-level range of motion (ROM) or calisthenic exercise, slow walking, or low intensity swimming can have a beneficial effect on physiologic function and other fitness factors that help maintain one's ability to perform activities of daily living (ADL) and enhance the quality of life.

ACSM's STATEMENT ON EXERCISE

The American College of Sports Medicine's (ACSM) position statement on the recommended quantity and quality of exercise for developing and maintaining fitness in healthy adults (American College of Sports Medicine, in press) makes the following recommendations for developing and maintaining cardiorespiratory fitness, body composition, and muscular strength and endurance in healthy adults: (a) Frequency of training should be 3–5 days per week. (b) Intensity of training should be 50–85% of maximum oxygen uptake ($\dot{V}O_2max$) or maximum heart rate (HRmax) reserve. (c) Duration of training should be 20–60 minutes of continuous aerobic activity, depending on the intensity of the activity; lower intensity activity should be conducted over a longer period of time. Because of the importance of the ''total fitness'' effect and the fact that this effect is more readily obtained in longer duration programs, and because of the potential hazards and compliance problems associated with high intensity activity, lower to moderate intensity activity of longer duration is recommended for nonathletic adults. (d)

The mode of activity can be any activity that uses large muscle groups, can be maintained continuously, and is rhythmical and aerobic in nature such as walking–hiking, running–jogging, cycling–bicycling, cross-country skiing, dancing, rope skipping, rowing, stair climbing, swimming, skating, and various endurance game activities. (e) Resistance training of moderate intensity sufficient to develop and maintain fat free weight (FFW) and bone integrity should be an integral part of an adult fitness program. Eight to 10 exercises that condition the major muscle groups at least 2 days per week is the recommended minimum.

EXERCISE GUIDELINES FOR THE ELDERLY

Do these same guidelines and standards for exercise prescription relate to the elderly? Certainly the improvement of physical fitness should be an important consideration in designing exercise programs for the elderly, but for many, enhancing the ability to perform daily living activities and/or improving and maintaining the quality of life will be the most important goal. In general, many of the basic guidelines for exercise prescription that have been developed for the middle-aged population are appropriate for the elderly.

The biggest difference would be in the application of the exercise prescription (Lampman, 1987; Pollock & Wilmore, in press; Wheat, 1987). The elderly participant is more fragile and thus more susceptible to fatigue, orthopedic injury, and possible cardiovascular problems (Larson & Bruce, 1987; Pollock & Wilmore, in press). Thus the exercise prescription for the elderly will include activities that are of low impact, that is, activities that produce less impact force on the musculoskeletal/joint structure (American College of Sports Medicine, in press). Also the prescription will be performed at a more moderate intensity and be applied in a more gradual fashion (Lampman, 1987; Morse & Smith, 1981; Pollock & Wilmore, in press; Wheat, 1987). In other words, the progression of the program should be slower to allow a more gradual adaptation to the training program.

Components of an Exercise Program

The components of a training program for the elderly participant would be similar to those recommended for the young and middle-aged adult (Pollock & Wilmore, in press). The program would include warm-up, muscular conditioning, aerobics, and cool-down periods. It has been our experience that the total program should not last more than 1 hour (Pollock, 1988; Pollock & Wilmore, in press). Programs of longer duration usually have higher dropout rates. Thus one should design a program that includes all the basic components of a training program and takes into consideration the participant's individual needs and goals.

With the elderly participant, more emphasis would be placed on the warm-up and cool-down periods. The muscular conditioning period could come before or after the endurance aerobic period, depending on personal preference. The warm-up would include stretching, low-level calisthenics, and low-level aerobic activity such as slow walking, cycling, or swimming. The muscular conditioning period should include a higher level calisthenic and/or resistance training. The aerobic period could include a variety of endurance activities such as fast walking, swimming, cycling, or rowing.

Low-impact aerobic endurance activity should be emphasized, and more will be said about this later. The cool-down should also include low-level aerobic activity such as slower walking, cycling, and stretching activities. The warm-up component should be conducted for 10 to 15 minutes and the cool-down for 5 to 10 minutes. The muscular conditioning period may take up to 15 or 20 minutes and aerobics from 30 to 45 minutes. Because of the time element, the muscular conditioning and aerobic periods may be conducted on alternate days, or certain aspects of these components can be emphasized on different days, thus minimizing the physical and time demands.

A well-rounded stretching and muscle conditioning period is recommended for all age groups (Cureton, 1969; Pollock & Wilmore, in press). It becomes even more important as we age because a loss of muscle mass and functional capacity of various body segments becomes quite apparent (Åstrand & Rodahl, 1986; Eckert & Montoye, 1983; Forbes, 1976; Smith & Serfass, 1981). For example, Pollock, Foster, Knapp, Rod, and Schmidt (1987) completed a 10-year follow-up study on masters runners whose ages ranged from 50 to 82 years. The study was designed to assess the runners' ability to maintain their aerobic capacity over a 10-year time span. Eleven of the 25 subjects evaluated continued to train at the same level over the 10-year period, and their aerobic capacity did not change (54.2 vs. 53.3 ml $\cdot$ kg^{-1} $\cdot$ min^{-1}), whereas the group who significantly reduced their training had a 10% decrease in aerobic capacity (52.5 vs. 45.9 ml $\cdot$ kg^{-1} $\cdot$ min^{-1}). These findings help to confirm the fact that reduction in aerobic capacity with age is lifestyle related (Buskirk & Hodgson, 1987; Hagberg, 1987; Kasch, Wallace, Van Camp, & Verity, 1988).

The striking finding in the investigation of masters runners was the significant loss in fat free weight (FFW) in both groups. The subjects as a whole showed a slight loss in total body weight with age and increase in body fat, and on the average showed a 2.0 kg decline in FFW over this time span. Considering their low body fat (13.2%) and continued training, this was a surprising loss. Short-term studies with younger individuals showed that FFW is usually maintained or increased with training (Pollock & Jackson, 1977; Pollock & Wilmore, in press). Also, weight/resistance training activities generally increase muscle mass, whereas aerobic activities maintain it (Berger, 1963; Fleck & Kraemer, 1987; Gettman & Pollock, 1981; Gillam, 1981; Misner, Boileau, Massey, & Mayhew, 1974; Wilmore, 1974).

Although aging is an important factor, it probably was not the only factor that caused the significant loss of FFW in these masters runners. It is thought that the manner in which they trained also contributed to the loss of FFW. It is well known that the training mode has a significant specificity effect on the training results (Åstrand & Rodahl, 1986), that is, arm training more specifically affects the arms, and leg training affects the legs. The specificity factor was supported by the circumference measures taken of the biceps (arm) and thigh. The biceps girth showed a significant reduction while the thigh remained constant.

An interview with each athlete revealed that most of them only trained aerobically and only occasionally, if at all, did stretching or strength training activities. Of interest was that 3 of the 25 subjects did significant upper-body training as part of their regular regimen. Two weight trained and one was an avid cross-country skier and participated in this activity 4 months a year. These three athletes were the only ones who maintained their FFW. Age did not seem to be a factor since there was one athlete for each decade of age from 50 to 80 years. More research concerning the effect of strength training on the long-term maintenance of FFW is necessary before a definitive statement can be made. These data illustrate the importance of specificity of training and the need for a well-rounded exercise program that includes not only aerobics but also stretching and muscular conditioning of all the major muscle groups of the body.

Although calisthenics can provide enough overload to produce increases in strength in low fit individuals, higher intensity resistance training may be necessary for a large percentage of the healthy, elderly population (Marcinik, Hodgdon, Mittleman, & O'Brien, 1985; Smith, Reddan, & Smith, 1981; Suominen, Heikkinen, & Tarkatti, 1977). The development of new equipment such as variable resistance exercise devices makes this type of training particularly suitable and safe for the elderly population (Wescott, 1987). The following are some advantages of the resistance training machines:

1. Weight (intensity) can be applied at a low level and can be increased in small increments.
2. Most of the equipment is built to protect the lower back, thus the potential for injury is lessened.
3. The variable resistance is advantageous and allows the stimulus to be applied more evenly through the full ROM.
4. Many exercise devices are designed to avoid the handgrip maneuver. This is important because handgripping can cause dramatic increases in blood pressure during exercise (Lind & McNicol, 1967).
5. Much of the equipment can be double pinned so that the subject's range of motion can be limited. This is particularly important in elderly participants who have arthritis and other joint problems. Thus the elderly participants can be exercised within the range of motion at which they do not experience discomfort or pain. It has been shown that limited range of motion exercise can still provide full range benefits to a training program (Graves, Pollock, Jones, Colvin, & Leggett, in press).

Even though resistance training may be appropriate and recommended for elderly participants, the recommendation would still call for moderation. Although the purpose of the muscular conditioning period is strength development, the maintenance of functional capacity and FFW would be equally important.

Endurance Training:
Low-Impact and Moderate Intensity Activities

The aerobic endurance training period will differ from the prescription designed for young to middle-age adults relative to intensity. The recommended intensity of exercise would be more moderate, and thus emphasis would be placed on added duration and frequency of training (American College of Sports Medicine, in press; Lampman, 1987; Pollock & Wilmore, in press; Wheat, 1987). The lower intensity exercise would help participants avoid injuries that are closely related to high-intensity programs and avoid potential cardiovascular events (Pollock, 1988; Pollock, Gettman, et al., 1978; Waller, 1987).

More important, because of the strong relationship between high-impact activities and injuries, low-impact activities should be emphasized (Kilbom et al., 1969; Mann et al., 1969; Oja, Teraslinna, Partanen, & Karava, 1974; Pollock, Gettman, et al., 1977; Richie, Kelso, & Bellucci, 1985). The data presented in Table 1 show the difference in injury rates of participants of various ages engaged in a 5- to 6-month training program of walking (W) and walking/jogging (W/J) conducted for 30 to 40 minutes, 3 (W/J) to 4 (W) days per week (Pollock et al., 1976; Pollock et al., 1977; Pollock, Hagberg, Graves, Leggett, S., Limacher, & Thomas, 1988; Pollock et al., 1971). All subjects were healthy, sedentary volunteers.

Table 1

Comparison of Injuries by Age

Study	N	Age range	Mode	Injuries (%)
Pollock et al., 1977	50	20–35	W/J	18
Pollock et al., 1976	22	49–65	W/J	41
Pollock et al., 1988	14	70–79	W/J	57
Pollock et al., 1971	19	40–56	W	12

Note. All programs were conducted with healthy previously sedentary individuals. Except for Pollock et al. (1971), all programs had a walk/jog (W/J) component. The 1971 study included only walking (W) as the mode of training. Injuries occurred mainly in the foot, ankle, leg, or knee and were associated with nonparticipation for at least 1 week.

In the earlier experiments (Pollock et al., 1976; Pollock et al., 1977), training began with equal amounts of W/J and progressed to more continuous jogging as adaptation to training occurred. In our recent investigation (Pollock et al., 1988), jogging was not introduced until after 3 months of moderate paced walking (50–60% HRmax reserve, rating of perceived exertion [RPE] 11–12) to fast walking (60–70% HRmax reserve, RPE 12–13) training. It is obvious from Table 1 that injuries are related to age and the high-impact forces produced by jogging.

It was surprising that even after 3 months of preliminary training the injury rate would be so high when the 70-year-old subjects began to walk/jog. The injuries occurred immediately during the first week of W/J, and in all cases but one were resolved within 3 weeks of training on a stationary cycle or slow walking on a treadmill. One woman had a stress fracture of the tibia and could not continue in the study. Eventually all of the 70–79-year-old subjects could get their training heart rate to 75–85% HRmax reserve (RPE = 14 to 15). The injured subjects continued to walk on the treadmill at an elevation that elicited the desired heart rate response. The total group had a 22% increase in $\dot{V}O_2max$, thus with these healthy 70-year-olds the prescribed program (W/J) was not limited by their cardiorespiratory system/capacity but by their musculoskeletal system (orthopedic limitations).

The fast walking program shown in Table 1 (Pollock et al., 1971) produced a 30% increase in $\dot{V}O_2$max and had the lowest injury (12%) and dropout rate of any of the 20 endurance training studies conducted by Pollock and colleagues since 1968. These data (Pollock et al., 1971) and others have clearly shown that walking is an effective program for developing aerobic fitness and improving body composition (Leon, Conrad, Hunninghake, & Serfass, 1979; Pollock, Dimmick, Miller, Kendrick, & Linnerud, 1975; Sharkey & Holleman, 1967). The trade-off with walking programs compared to jogging is the need to increase the frequency and duration of training. Walking is simplistic in nature and requires little in terms of skill, facilities, and equipment. Its lower intensity and impact forces make it safe and easily adaptable to elderly participants.

Table 2 lists commonly used high- and low-impact activities for developing and maintaining aerobic endurance. The big distinction among activities is whether or not they cause high-impact forces on the joints. Any activity that has a running and/or jumping component is considered a high-impact type of activity. The inclusion of high-impact and high-intensity activities into a program in combination with high frequency and duration increases the injury rate exponentially (Blair, Kohl, & Goodyear, 1987; Mann et al., 1969; Oja et al., 1974; Pollock et al., 1977; Powell, Kohl, Caspersen, & Blair, 1986; Richie et al., 1985). Thus, when considering an aerobic training program, activities or regimens that are associated with higher injury rates should be avoided.

Using RPE to Monitor Intensity of Training

Training intensity is usually determined by calculating a heart rate value that corresponds to a percent of maximum heart rate. The training zone for developing and maintaining fitness ranges from 50 to 85% of HRmax reserve (American College of Sports Medicine, in press; Pollock & Wilmore, in press). More recently, the RPE scale developed by Borg (1982; Borg & Ottoson, 1986) has been used to help monitor training intensity (American College of Sports Medicine, in press; Birk & Birk, 1987; Pollock, Jackson, & Foster, 1986; Pollock & Wilmore, in press). The RPE scale relates well to both oxygen uptake and heart rate

Table 2

Commonly Used High-Impact and Low-Impact Activities for Aerobic Endurance Training

High-impact	Low-impact
Jogging/running	Walking
Basketball/volleyball	Cycling-bicycling
Hopping/jogging activities	Swimming/water activities
Rope skipping	Rowing
Aerobic dance (high-impact)	Stair climbing
	Aerobic dance (low-impact)
	Cross-country skiing

(Borg, 1982; Borg & Ottoson, 1986). Thus, the knowledge of both heart rate and RPE will allow the participant to regulate his or her training program physiologically and perceptually. Exercising at an intensity that produces a training effect is important, and at the same time, regulating the program at a perceptually acceptable level (moderate to somewhat hard) will aid in long-term adherence.

Classification of Exercise Intensity

Is the training intensity for exercise prescription calculated and interpreted in the same manner for elderly participants as for young and middle-aged adults? In our experience with elderly healthy subjects and cardiac patients the answer is yes (Pollock et al., 1976; Pollock et al., 1988; Pollock et al., 1986). Table 3 shows a recommended classification of exercise intensity based on endurance exercise programs lasting 30–60 minutes (Pollock & Wilmore, in press). The table lists the relationship between percent of HRmax reserve and RPE. Based on the elderly participants' individualized exercise test results, these markers of intensity have similar value and meaning in the training and the progression of training in the elderly as compared to younger participants. Although more research is needed to provide the necessary guidelines for developing programs for long-term adherence in the elderly, it appears that "somewhat hard," 12–13 on the RPE scale, is an appropriate recommendation for the maintenance of aerobic fitness, body composition, and muscular strength and endurance.

Progression of Endurance Training

Information concerning the progression of training in the elderly is lacking in the literature. Most studies allude to a longer, more gradual adaptation period, but precise quantification is absent. In 1978 Pollock, Wilmore, and Fox suggested that a 40% increase in time should be allowed for adaptation to training for each decade of life after age 30. Thus, if 30-year-old participants progress every

Table 3

Classification of Intensity of Exercise Based on 30 to 60 Minutes of Endurance Training

Relative intensity $\dot{V}O_2$max or HRmax reserve	Rating of perceived exertion	Classification of intensity
< 30%	< 10	Very light
30–49%	10–11	Light
50–74%	12–13	Moderate
75–84%	14–16	Heavy
> 85%	> 16	Very heavy

Note. Table adapted from Pollock & Wilmore, in press, *Exercise in Health and Disease: Evaluation and Prescription for Prevention and Rehabilitation* (2nd ed.). Philadelphia: Saunders.

week, then 50-year-olds will progress every 2 weeks and 70-year-olds every 3 to 4 weeks. Although this approximation of the time needed for various age groups to progress in training has worked fairly well, it has not been adequately tested. Also, because the increment in progression from one step to another is usually smaller in older and more fragile participants, the 40% rule suggested above may not be an appropriate standard. For an alternative, if elderly participants are rating their training at 10–11 (fairly light) on the RPE scale then weekly increases in training load will be acceptable. If/when exercise is perceived at 12–13 (somewhat hard), then progression will be slower, perhaps every 2–3 weeks.

Program Modifications for the Elderly

A final point on the mode of activity used for training is particularly appropriate for the elderly. Many elderly persons have special physical–medical problems that cause poor vision, an unsteady gait, and/or musculoskeletal limitations. As a result of these problems the exercise specialist has to be particularly careful in getting the participant into the proper activity (Wheat, 1987). Lack of understanding of physical–medical problems and/or delay in having pertinent records available when starting the program could lead to an avoidable injury or a bad experience. Initial individual counseling and program monitoring will help avoid major problems.

SUMMARY

The needs and goals of an exercise program for a healthy and ambulatory elderly person emphasizes fitness development, but the maintenance of functional capacity and quality of life are equally important. The basic guidelines of frequency, intensity, and duration of training and mode of activity recommended by the American College of Sports Medicine for healthy adults are also appropriate for the elderly. The big difference in the exercise prescription for the elderly participant is the manner in which it is applied.

Usually, given that the elderly person is more fragile and has more physical–medical limitations than the middle-aged participant, the intensity of the program is lower when training frequency and duration are increased. The mode of training should avoid high-impact activities, and progression of training should be more gradual. The calculation of the training heart rate, 50–85% of HRmax reserve, and its relationship to relative metabolic work and rating of perceived exertion are similar to those found for younger participants. Because of the importance of maintaining muscle mass and bone in middle and old age, a well-rounded program including strength/resistance exercise of the major muscle groups is recommended. Hence the exercise prescription for the elderly will emphasize low- to moderate-intensity and low-impact activities, avoid heavy static–dynamic lifting, and allow for a slow, gradual adaptation period.

REFERENCES

AMERICAN College of Sports Medicine. (in press). The recommended quantity and quality of exercise for developing and maintaining fitness in healthy adults (2nd ed.). *Medicine and Science in Sports and Exercise*.

ÅSTRAND, P.O., & Rodahl, K. (1986). *Textbook of work physiology* (3rd ed.). New York: McGraw-Hill.

BADENHOP, D.T., Cleary, P.A., Schaal, S.F., Fox, E.L., & Bartels, R.L. (1983). Physiological adjustments to higher- or lower-intensity exercise in elders. *Medicine and Science in Sports and Exercise,* **15**, 496-502.

BARRY, A.J., Daly, J.W., Pruett, E.D.R., Steinmetz, J.R., Page, H.F., Birkhead, N.C., & Rodahl, K. (1966). The effects of physical conditioning on older individuals. I. Work capacity, circulatory–respiratory function, and work electrocardiogram. *Journal of Gerontology,* **21**, 182-191.

BERGER, R.A. (1963). Comparative effects of three weight training programs. *Research Quarterly,* **34**, 396-398.

BIRK, T.J., & Birk, C.A. (1987). Use of ratings of perceived exertion for exercise prescription. *Journal of Sports Medicine,* **4**, 1-8.

BLAIR, S.N., Kohl, H.W., & Goodyear, N.N. (1987). Rates and risks for running and exercise injuries: Studies in three populations. *Research Quarterly for Exercise and Sport,* **58**, 221-228.

BORG, G.A.V. (1982). Psychophysical bases of perceived exertion. *Medicine and Science in Sports and Exercise,* **14**, 377-381.

BORG, G., & Ottoson, D. (1986). *The perception of exertion in physical work.* London: Macmillan Press.

BUSKIRK, E.R., & Hodgson, J.S. (1987). Age and aerobic power: The rate of change in men and women. *Federation Proceedings,* **46**, 1824-1829.

CURETON, T.K. (1969). *The physiological effects of exercise programs on adults.* Springfield, IL: Charles C Thomas.

DeVRIES, H.A. (1970). Physiological effects of an exercise training regimen upon men aged 52–88. *Journal of Gerontology,* **25**, 325-336.

ECKERT, H.M., & Montoye, H.J. (Eds.) (1983). *The Academy Papers, No. 17. Exercise and health.* Champaign, IL: Human Kinetics.

FLECK, S.J., & Kraemer, W.J. (1987). *Designing resistance training programs.* Champaign, IL: Human Kinetics.

FORBES, G.B. (1976). The adult decline in lean body mass. *Human Biology,* **48**, 161-173.

GETTMAN, L.R., & Pollock, M.L. (1981). Circuit weight training: A critical review of its physiological benefits. *The Physician and Sportsmedicine,* **9**, 44-60.

GILLAM, G.M. (1981). Effects of frequency of weight training on muscle strength enhancement. *Journal of Sports Medicine,* **21**, 432-436.

GRAVES, J.E., Pollock, M.L., Jones, A.E., Colvin, A.B., & Leggett, S.H. (in press). Specificity of limited range of motion variable resistance training. *Medicine and Science in Sports and Exercise.*

HAGBERG, J.M. (1987). Effect of training on the decline of $\dot{V}O_2$max with aging. *Federation Proceedings,* **46**, 1830-1833.

KASCH, F.W., Wallace, J.P., Van Camp, S.P., & Verity, L. (1988). A longitudinal study of cardiovascular stability in active men aged 45–65 years. *The Physician and Sportsmedicine, 16,* 117-124.

KILBOM, A., Hartley, L.H., Saltin, B., Bjure, J., Grimby, G., & Åstrand, I. (1969). Physical training in sedentary middle-aged and older men. *Scandinavian Journal of Clinical and Laboratory Investigation, 24,* 315-322.

LAMPMAN, R.M. (1987). Evaluating and prescribing exercise for elderly patients. *Geriatrics, 42,* 63-73.

LARSON, E.B., & Bruce, R.A. (1987). Health benefits of exercise in an aging society. *Archives of Internal Medicine, 147,* 353-356.

LEON, A.S., Conrad, J., Hunninghake, D.B., & Serfass, R. (1979). Effects of a vigorous walking program on body composition, and carbohydrate and lipid metabolism of obese young men. *American Journal of Clinical Nutrition, 32,* 1776-1787.

LIND, A.R., & McNicol, G. (1967). Muscular factors which determine the cardiovascular responses to sustained and rhythmic exercise. *Canadian Medical Association Journal, 96,* 706-713.

MANN, G.V., Garrett, L.H., Farhi, A., Murray, H., Billings, T.F., Shute, F., & Schwarten, S.E. (1969). Exercise to prevent coronary heart disease. *American Journal of Medicine, 46,* 12-27.

MARCINIK, E.J., Hodgdon, J.A., Mittleman, K., & O'Brien, J.J. (1985). Aerobic/calisthenic and aerobic/circuit weight training programs for Navy men: A comparative study. *Medicine and Science in Sports and Exercise, 17,* 482-487.

MISNER, J.E., Boileau, R.A., Massey, B.H., & Mayhew, J.L. (1974). Alterations in the body composition of adult men during selected physical training programs. *Journal of the American Geriatrics Society, 27,* 33-38.

MIYASHITA, M., Haga, S., & Mitzuta, T. (1978). Training and detraining effects on aerobic power in middle-aged and older men. *Journal of Sports Medicine, 18,* 131-137.

MORSE, C.E., & Smith, E.L. (1981). Physical activity programming for the aged. In E.L. Smith & R.C. Serfass (Eds.), *Exercise and aging: The scientific basis* (pp. 109-120). Hillside, NJ: Enslow.

OJA, P., Teraslinna, P., Partanen, T., & Karava, R. (1974). Feasibility of an 18 months' physical training program for middle-aged men and its effect on physical fitness. *American Journal of Public Health, 64,* 459-465.

POLLOCK, M.L. (1988). Prescribing exercise for fitness and adherence. In R.K. Dishman (Ed.), *Exercise adherence: Its impact on public health* (pp. 259-277). Champaign, IL: Human Kinetics.

POLLOCK, M.L., Dawson, G.A., Miller, H.S., Jr., Ward, A., Cooper, D., Headley, W., Linnerud, A.C., & Nomeir, M.M. (1976). Physiologic responses of men 49 to 65 years of age to endurance training. *Journal of the American Geriatrics Society, 24,* 97-104.

POLLOCK, M.L., Dimmick, J., Miller, H.S., Kendrick, Z., & Linnerud, A.C. (1975). Effects of mode of training on cardiovascular function and body composition of middle-aged men. *Medicine and Science in Sports, 7,* 139-145.

POLLOCK, M.L., Foster, C., Knapp, D., Rod, J.L., & Schmidt, D.H. (1987). Effect of age and training on aerobic capacity and body composition of master athletes. *Journal of Applied Physiology,* **62**, 725-731.

POLLOCK, M.L., Gettman, L.R., Milesis, C.A., Bah, M.D., Durstine, L., & Johnson, R.B. (1977). Effects of frequency and duration of training on attrition and incidence of injury. *Medicine and Science in Sports,* **9**, 31-36.

POLLOCK, M.L., Gettman, L.R., Raven, P.B., Ayres, J., Bah, M., & Ward, A. (1978). Physiological comparison of the effects of aerobic and anaerobic training. In C.S. Price, M.L. Pollock, L.R. Gettman, & D.A. Kent (Eds.), *Physical fitness programs for law enforcement officers: A manual for police administrators* (pp. 89-96). Washington, DC: U.S. Government Printing Office.

POLLOCK, M.L., Hagberg, J.M., Graves, J.E., Leggett, S., Limacher, M., & Thomas, W.C. (1988). *Injuries associated with walking, jogging and resistance training in 70-79-year-old men and women.* Unpublished manuscript.

POLLOCK, M.L., & Jackson, A. (1977). Body composition: Measurement and changes resulting from physical training. In L.I. Gedvilas & M.E. Kneer (Eds.), *Proceedings of the NCPEM/NAPECW National Conference* (pp. 125-136).

POLLOCK, M.L., Jackson, A.S., & Foster, C. (1986). The use of the perception scale for exercise prescription. In G. Borg & D. Ottoson, (Eds.), *The perception of exertion in physical work* (pp. 161-176). London: MacMillan.

POLLOCK, M.L., Miller, H., Janeway, R., Linnerud, A.C., Robertson, B., & Valentino, R. (1971). Effects of walking on body composition and cardiovascular function of middle-aged men. *Journal of Applied Physiology,* **30**, 126-130.

POLLOCK, M.L., & Wilmore, J. (in press). *Exercise in health and disease: Evaluation and prescription for prevention and rehabilitation* (2nd ed.). Philadelphia: Saunders.

POLLOCK, M.L., Wilmore, J.H., & Fox, S.M. (1978). *Health and fitness through physical activity.* New York: Wiley.

POWELL, K.E., Kohl, H.W., Caspersen, C.J., & Blair, S.N. (1986). An epidemiological perspective of the causes of running injuries. *The Physician and Sportsmedicine,* **14**, 100-114.

RICHIE, D.H., Kelso, S.F., & Bellucci, P.A. (1985). Aerobic dance injuries: A retrospective study of instructors and participants. *The Physician and Sportsmedicine,* **13**, 114-120.

SEALS, D.R., Hagberg, J.M., Hurley, B.F., Ehsani, A.A., & Holloszy, J.O. (1984). Endurance training in older men and women I. Cardiovascular responses to exercise. *Journal of Applied Physiology,* **57**, 1024-1029.

SHARKEY, B.J., & Holleman, J.P. (1967). Cardiorespiratory adaptations to training at specified intensities. *Research Quarterly,* **38**, 698-704.

SIDNEY, K.H., Shephard, R.J., & Harrison, J. (1977). Endurance training and body composition of the elderly. *American Journal of Clinical Nutrition,* **30**, 326-333.

SMITH, E.L., Reddan, W., & Smith, P.E. (1981). Physical activity and calcium modalities for bone mineral increase in aged women. *Medicine and Science in Sports and Exercise,* **13**, 60-64.

SMITH, E.L., & Serfass, R.C. (Eds.) (1981). *Exercise and aging: The scientific basis.* Hillside, NJ: Enslow.

SUOMINEN, H., Heikkinen, E., & Tarkatti, T. (1977). Effect of eight weeks physical training on muscle and connective tissue of the m. vastus lateralis in 69-year-old men and women. *Journal of Gerontology,* **32**, 33-37.

WALLER, B.F. (1987). Sudden death in middle-aged conditioned subjects: Coronary atherosclerosis is the culprit. *Mayo Clinical Proceedings,* **62**, 634-636.

WESCOTT, W.L. (1987). *Strength fitness: Physiological principles and training techniques* (2nd ed.). Boston: Allyn & Bacon.

WHEAT, M.E. (1987). Exercise in the elderly. *Western Journal of Medicine,* **147**, 477-480.

WILMORE, J.H. (1974). Alterations in strength, body composition, and anthropometric measurements to a 10-week weight training program. *Medicine and Science in Sports,* **6**, 133-138.

The Aging of Cardiovascular Function

Roy J. Shephard
University of Toronto

Until recently, the aging of cardiovascular function seemed a relatively simple process. The maximum steady-state oxygen intake showed a progressive, age-related decline, beginning around the age of 20 years (Shephard, 1978, 1987), and there was an associated progressive decline in the main determinant of maximum oxygen transport, the maximum cardiac output (Niinimaa & Shephard, 1978). Several factors have recently helped to complicate this analysis.

First, it has been argued that the decline in maximum oxygen intake with age, for all its apparent regularity in many different cross-sectional and longitudinal surveys, is sometimes at least partly an artifact of declining habitual activity (Heath, Hagberg, Ehsani, & Holloszy, 1981; Rode & Shephard, 1984). Second, some authors such as Lakatta, Mitchell, Pomerance, and Rowe (1987) have experienced difficulty in defining a satisfactory oxygen consumption plateau when testing elderly patients on the cycle ergometer, and they have argued from this observation that function may have been limited by difficulty in shunting cardiac output to the exercising limbs, a limited muscle mass, or some factor other than the pumping ability of the heart. Perhaps the most telling piece of new evidence was obtained on rigorously screened volunteers from the Baltimore longitudinal study of aging (Rodeheffer et al., 1984; Weisfeldt, Gerstenblith, & Lakatta, 1985). If subjects with ischemic changes in the myocardium were excluded by a combination of electrocardiography and scintigraphy, it was argued that the classical age-related decrease of maximum cardiac output was not observed; rather, the Frank-Starling mechanism was invoked, so that an increased end-diastolic volume and an increased maximum stroke volume compensated for the decline in maximal heart rate. The views of the Baltimore team have been widely publicized, and the time may thus be opportune to review these new concepts critically relative to classical views on cardiac aging.

AGE AND MAXIMUM OXYGEN INTAKE

The aging of maximum oxygen intake raises several distinct issues: (a) Can the rate of functional loss be inferred from changes in physical performance? (b) Can aerobic power be measured directly in the older person, and if so, what influence does habitual activity have on functional loss? (c) Is the maximum oxygen intake of an older subject limited by cardiac output, as in a younger person, and if not, what change is responsible for the impaired performance?

Inferences From Performance Data

The performance in many endurance events, including cross-country skiing, distance swimming, orienteering, and distance running, deteriorates regularly over the span of adult life (Rahe & Arthur, 1975; Riegel, 1981; Saltin, 1986; Stones & Kozma, 1980). In some sports, mechanical efficiency may deteriorate with aging, but there is probably little change in the mechanical efficiency of running; it is thus tempting to infer the rate of oxygen transport loss from the increase in record track times, about 1% per year of age in men. The weakness in this inference is that a constant level of competition is assumed at all ages, when in fact competition is much more keen among the younger age groups. The problem is highlighted by extending the analysis to women, whereby the increase of running times amounts to about 2.5% per year (Stones & Kozma, 1982). At best, an analysis of track performances can set an upper limit to the loss of aerobic power with aging.

Making Direct Maximum Oxygen Intake Measurements in the Elderly

Because of a commendable desire to obtain scintigraphic measurements of cardiac output, the recent studies of "maximum voluntary exercise" reported by Lakatta et al. (1987) have been made on a cycle ergometer. Even in young adults there are often difficulties in reaching a well-defined plateau of oxygen consumption on a cycle ergometer. Unless an older subject is a trained cyclist, a large part of his or her required muscular effort is sustained by a quadriceps muscle which has been weakened by aging and is contracting at a high percentage of its maximum voluntary force. The resultant external vascular impedance presents a prohibitive afterload to the heart, and effort is halted by a local accumulation of lactic acid before peak cardiac output has been realized (Kay & Shephard, 1969). Lakatta et al. (1987) do not cite figures for oxygen transport, but speak of difficulty in reaching a plateau. The peak heart rates illustrated in their graphs are all quite low relative to usually accepted population maxima for the age groups under investigation.

On the other hand, if treadmill testing is adopted, maximum oxygen intake can be measured successfully into the ninth decade of life (Sidney & Shephard, 1977a). Three quarters of elderly subjects show a classical oxygen consumption plateau at their first evaluation; in at least half of the remaining individuals, a plateau can be realized with a second attempt, and in the other subjects ancillary values such as heart rate, respiratory gas exchange ratio, and blood lactate concentrations are high enough to confirm that a true maximum effort has been realized. We may thus conclude that with an appropriate choice of methodology, it is generally possible to make a direct measurement of maximum oxygen intake in the healthy elderly person.

Habitual Activity and Age Changes in Maximum Oxygen Intake

The possible impact of changes in habitual activity upon the apparent rate of aging of maximum oxygen intake is not a new issue. Hollmann (1965) and Dehn and Bruce (1972) argued that the rate of functional loss was less in an athletic sample than in the general population. However, the figures they cited for athletes (an annual loss of 0.70 and 0.56 ml • kg⁻¹min⁻¹, respectively) did not differ substantially from the rate of loss seen by others who have tested the general population (Shephard, 1987). For example, longitudinal studies of physical education teachers by Asmussen and Mathiasen (1962) have shown a steady decline in aerobic power of some 5 ml • kg⁻¹min⁻¹ per decade.

One factor causing confusion has been the tendency of a functional evaluation to stimulate a previously sedentary population to adopt an active lifestyle. Thus, over a period of 10 years, it appeared to Kasch and Wallace (1976) that there had been no decline of maximum oxygen intake among men recruited to a vigorous exercise program; however, when the study was extended 5 more years, the normal slope of the aging process reappeared, although all maximum oxygen intake values were set at a higher level (Kasch & Kulberg, 1981).

Åstrand (1986) described a similar phenomenon. He studied four physical education students in 1949, 1970, and 1982; at the 1970 evaluation, all showed a classical loss of aerobic power, but in 1982 two of the subjects (who had trained very hard in preparation for their reevaluation) had restored maximum oxygen intake close to their 1949 scores. Heath et al. (1981) matched 16 masters athletes with 16 younger athletes on the basis of training miles, training intensity, and best performance at comparable ages. The maximum oxygen intake at an average age of 59 years was 58 ml • kg⁻¹ min⁻¹, and Heath et al. argued that if the functional loss in these individuals had been 9% per decade (as in their general cross-sectional studies), then values at age 25 years would have averaged 81 ml • kg⁻¹ min¹ rather than the 69 ml • kg⁻¹ min⁻¹ observed in the young athletes. They thus suggested that active subjects had lost only 5% of function per decade, an amount that could be attributed simply to the decline in maximum heart rate. It should be stressed here that part of the argument is semantic, since other authors have attributed to athletes the same absolute and not the same percentage decline in function as that seen in sedentary individuals.

Kavanagh and Shephard (1977) were able to verify the average training distance in a sample of masters competitors. Figures were almost identical for the youngest category (average age 34.8 years) and those aged 60–70 years, with a decline in aerobic power of only 2.8 ml • kg⁻¹ min⁻¹ per decade over a 28.8-year age span. Training distances were also similar for the groups aged 40–50 and 50–60 years, with a decrease in maximum oxygen intake of 3.8 ml • kg⁻¹ min⁻¹ over a 10.3-year age span.

These figures, which have recently been confirmed by the same authors in a much larger sample of masters athletes, agree quite closely with the loss of 3.2 ml • kg⁻¹ min⁻¹ hypothesized by Heath et al. (1981). Likewise, Pollock et al. (1974) found equivalent training distances in masters competitors at 40–50 and 50–60 years of age, but nevertheless the aerobic power of the latter group was 3.1 ml • kg⁻¹ min⁻¹ smaller. In contrast, Saltin (1986) described a loss of 7.3 ml • kg⁻¹ min⁻¹ in still-active orienteers. There are three possible explanations of this conflicting finding: (a) the initial aerobic power of Saltin's group was much higher (81 ml • kg⁻¹ min⁻¹ as young adults), (b) the age span studied by Saltin was later (from about 55 to 75 years), and (c) possible changes in the weekly training distance of orienteers were not verified (although the best competitors were said to have increased their weekly distance as they became older).

We may thus conclude that if the activity of the subject is held constant, the loss of aerobic power among continuing athletes is somewhat less than in the general population (whose habitual activity is progressively declining); nevertheless it amounts to somewhere between 2.8 and 3.8 ml • kg⁻¹ min⁻¹ per decade, a loss of 5 to 6%.

Determinants of Maximum Oxygen Intake

In some older people, the subject or the supervising physician halts effort short of a traditional oxygen consumption plateau because of breathlessness, anginal pain, or alarming electrocardiographic appearances rather than a limitation of cardiac output (Gerstenblith, Lakatta, & Weisfeldt, 1976; Jones, 1984). However, the usually reported reasons for halting a progressive exercise test (a feeling of weakness in the muscles, poor coordination, or impending loss of consciousness) seem expressions of an inadequate cardiac output rather than respiratory failure. With a typical maximum test protocol, breathlessness does not become severe until 2–4 minutes after exercise has ceased, as lactic acid diffusing out of the active muscles begins to affect the respiratory centers.

Nevertheless, manifestations of myocardial ischemia (anginal pain, premature ventricular contractions, and deep ST segmental depression) limit oxygen transport in some subjects over the age of 40 years. By the age of 65 years, 30% of sedentary patients develop symptoms or signs that lead many physicians to abort a maximum exercise test (Montoye, 1975; Sidney & Shephard, 1977b). The regular endurance exercise undertaken by many masters athletes reduces myocardial oxygen demand (since the pulse-pressure product is lower at any given external power output) and it also improves coronary perfusion (since the diastolic phase of the cardiac cycle is relatively longer than in the sedentary individual). However, these theoretical advantages tend to be lost during maximal effort, and in practice the proportion of masters athletes with abnormal exercise ECG records is much as in sedentary subjects (Kavanagh & Shephard, 1977).

In a recent large-scale survey of older competitors, we found 10.9% of abnormalities in those aged 30–39, and in subsequent decades 13.8, 20.4, 27.5, and 29.6% of electrocardiographic (ECG) records were abnormal (Kavanagh & Shephard, in preparation). Grimby and Saltin (1966) and Gibbons, Cooper, Martin, and Pollock (1977) have also found exercise ECG abnormalities in some 25% of masters athletes. Although myocardial ischemia limits performance in 20–25% of older competitors, we may conclude that in the remaining 75–80% oxygen intake is limited by maximal cardiac output.

AGE AND CARDIAC FUNCTION

If oxygen transport is indeed limited by maximal cardiac output, this may be calculated as the product of maximal heart rate, maximal arterio-venous oxygen difference, and maximal stroke volume. We shall thus look at the influence of age upon each of these variables in active subjects, considering also the implications for myocardial function.

Heart Rate

In the sedentary adult, the maximum heart rate declines from about 195 beats • min⁻¹ at the age of 25 years to around 170 beats • min⁻¹ at the age of 65 years (Shephard, 1977; Sidney & Shephard, 1977a), a loss of some 6.3% per decade.

Training is thought to induce some decrease in maximum heart rate, but nevertheless the effect of conditioning remains similar at different ages, so that the rate of decrease of heart rate with age is similar for the sedentary person, the average performer, and the top athlete (Saltin, 1986).

Arterio-Venous Oxygen Difference

There seems general agreement that, relative to the young adult, the arterio-venous oxygen difference of a sedentary older person is normal or even increased in submaximal effort, but the maximum arterio-venous oxygen difference is reduced by about 10% (Niinimaa & Shephard, 1978; Shephard, 1987). The elderly are not generally anemic, and the arterial oxygen content is usually well maintained, although it may decrease in subjects with a large maximum oxygen intake (Dempsey, 1987). The muscle capillarity of older orienteers (2–5 capillaries per muscle fiber) also remains much as in young athletes (2.7/fiber) and much more than in sedentary subjects (1.3–1.4/fiber). Likewise, mitochondrial enzyme activity is decreased by only 10–15% in older subjects. Saltin (1986) found a femoral venous oxygen content of only 18 ml $\cdot$ l^{-1} in elderly orienteers, compared with 25 ml $\cdot$ l^{-1} in their younger peers. Since problems of both oxygenation and extraction can be eliminated, the narrowed overall arterio-venous oxygen difference of the older adult must reflect a partial failure to redirect blood flow from the inactive muscles, viscera, and skin to the working tissue (Shephard, 1987). This is probably due in turn to a reduction of arterial elasticity and less ready vasodilatation of vessels in the active muscles (Saltin, 1986).

Skeletal muscle mass is better preserved against aging in the well-trained athlete, and because of a lesser thickness of subcutaneous fat and more ready sweating, there is less need to direct blood flow to the skin during exercise. However, the advantages of the trained person are more important during prolonged submaximal effort than in maximum exercise; Grimby, Nilsson, and Saltin (1966) and Saltin (1986) have all observed a relatively low maximum arterio-venous oxygen difference (134 ml $\cdot$ l^{-1}) in older orienteers.

In 1981, Heath et al. claimed that in distance runners the oxygen pulse (the product of arterio-venous oxygen difference and stroke volume) did not decline with age. If their inference from cross-sectional data is correct, it would suggest that any reduction of arterio-venous oxygen difference is compensated by an increase of stroke volume. Two weaknesses of this study were pointed out by Saltin (1986): To judge from maximum oxygen intakes, the young comparison group were not elite performers; and since exercise blood pressures were no higher in the older than in the younger group, it is debatable whether the former reached a true maximum effort (at which stroke volume might have been impaired by an increase of afterload).

Hagberg et al. revised their opinion in 1985, their later report suggesting a small decline of oxygen pulse with age. Saltin (1986) also found an age-related decline of oxygen pulse in orienteers, from 0.42 ml $\cdot$ kg^{-1} $\cdot$ $beat^{-1}$ at 26 years to 0.32 ml $\cdot$ kg^{-1} $\cdot$ $beat^{-1}$ at the age of 66 years, the 23.8% change reflecting both a decrease of arterio-venous oxygen difference and a decrease of maximum stroke volume. Even in the six best orienteers, who were actually increasing their training schedule, there was an age-related decrease of both maximum oxygen intake and oxygen pulse, the final figure of 0.32 ml $\cdot$ kg^{-1} $\cdot$ $beat^{-1}$ being much as for the group as a whole.

Stroke Volume

Lakatta et al. (1987) have argued that much of the supposed deterioration of cardiac function with age is due to subclinical disease. In the Baltimore study, if subjects with ischemic changes in the myocardium were excluded by a combination of electrocardiography and scintigraphy, then the classical age-related decrease of maximum cardiac output was not seen. Rather, the Frank-Starling mechanism was invoked, so that an increased end-diastolic volume and an increased maximum stroke volume compensated for the decline of maximum heart rate and maximum arterio-venous oxygen difference.

Certainly, severe myocardial ischemia can cause a decline of stroke volume (Parker, diGiorgi, & West, 1966), but it is less clear than the moderate ECG changes seen in 25% of older athletes have such an effect. Moreover, the concept of a population that is entirely free of subclinical ischemia seems somewhat artificial for the retirement years. The data for the Baltimore study show considerable scatter, and for technical reasons Lakatta et al. (1987) were unable to take their subjects to the usually accepted criteria of maximum performance (where a restriction of stroke volume might still have been observed). The maximum cardiac outputs for the younger age group also appear relatively low, whereas if the reported stroke volumes of the elderly subjects are multiplied by the usually accepted maximum heart rates for the elderly, the resultant cardiac outputs would require either an unrealistically large maximum oxygen intake or an unrealistically low arterio-venous oxygen difference. Unfortunately, Lakatta et al. (1987) provided no information on either of these variables. Finally, although the adverse effect of age upon the exercise-related increase of cardiac ejection fraction (Port, Cobb, Coleman, & Jones, 1980; Shocken, Blumenthal, Port, Hindle, & Coleman, 1983) is less marked after exclusion of patients with myocardial ischemia, it is not abolished; indeed, in many healthy subjects aged 60–80 years the ejection fraction during maximum exercise shows little or no increase over the resting ejection fraction (Rodeheffer et al., 1984).

Grimby and Saltin (1966; 1971) found that in 51-year-old orienteers, the maximum cardiac output was 5.1 • min^{-1} (17%) lower than in their 25-year-old peers. While much of this difference was due to a decrease of maximal heart rate, there was also a small decrease in plateau values for maximal stroke volume. More recent data on oxygen pulse in older competitors (Saltin, 1986) support this view, although it remains arguable that at least a part of the observed decrease in stroke volume of aging athletes is due to a decline in their training schedules.

It is well documented that the mean systemic blood pressure rises progressively with age, both at rest and during exercise (Hanson, Tabakin, Levy, & Nedde, 1968). Moreover, while there is some evidence that regular training can induce a therapeutically useful decrease of resting blood pressure (Tipton, 1984), during maximum effort well-trained subjects develop a larger cardiac output and thus as high a final blood pressure as their sedentary counterparts (Saltin, 1986). If the maximum stroke volume is well maintained in the face of this increased pressure, there must therefore be adaptive changes in the myocardium.

Myocardial Adaptations

An early autopsy report from Germany (Linzbach & Akuamoa-Boateng, 1973) suggested that heart mass increased between the ages of 30 and 90 years, by 1 g • yr^{-1} in men and 1.5 g • yr^{-1} in women; these changes are relatively small in a total mass of 350–400 g, but nevertheless match the usual age-dependent rise in resting blood pressure. Some early studies suggested that the radiographic heart shadow diminished with aging, but Kavanagh and Shephard (1977) found that in masters athletes the volume per unit of body mass was sustained and possibly even increased in older members of their sample. Likewise, echocardiographic data show a moderate age-related increase of left ventricular wall thickness in both systole and diastole (Gerstenblith et al., 1977; Nishimura, Yamada, & Kawai, 1980; Sjogren, 1971). The increase of cardiac mass seems due largely to an increase in average myocyte size (Unverferth, Fetters, & Unverferth, 1983), although there is also some accumulation of both collagen and amyloid (Hodkinson & Pomerance, 1977). It is less clearly established that the increase of cardiac mass increases maximum stroke volume. During peak effort, function could be adversely influenced by a decrease of preloading, an increase of afterloading, or a decrease of ventricular power.

Preloading

Structural deteriorations in the venous system, including varicosities, together with a decrease of total blood volume and poor tone in the capacity vessels, tend to reduce preloading for the sedentary older person. These problems are exacerbated by a decrease of ventricular compliance, with delayed relaxation in early diastole (Gerstenblith et al., 1977; Lakatta, 1980). Regular endurance activity tends to correct the situation by increasing total blood volume and increasing the tone of the peripheral veins; it is unclear whether continued training facilitates ventricular relaxation, but in some instances a powerful atrial contraction may also speed late diastolic filling (Lakatta, 1980).

Afterloading

With aging, afterloading is increased because a greater volume of blood must be accelerated in a distended aorta, and the arterial walls are less distensible (O'Rourke, 1982). As maximum effort is approached, atrophied muscles are forced to contract at a large fraction of their maximum voluntary force, and systemic blood pressure rises in an attempt to sustain their perfusion (Kay & Shephard, 1969). To the extent that regular training develops muscular strength, it may reverse one element of increased afterloading. There is also some potential to compensate for the increased arterial impedance through left ventricular hypertrophy, as already discussed.

Myocardial Contractility

Much of the increase of stroke volume that occurs during exercise is mediated by an increase of myocardial contractility. With aging, there is a decrease of beta-receptor sensitivity or density, reducing the inotropic response of the myocytes to a standard dose of catecholamine (Lakatta, 1980). It is unclear how far this is counteracted by an increase of circulating catecholamine levels during maximum exercise. In the rat, the aging heart muscle takes longer to develop peak force (Spurgeon, Steinbach, & Lakatta, 1983), and the indirect evidence of lengthened systolic time intervals suggests that a similar change occurs in older humans; a slowing of Ca^{2+} sequestration by the sarcoplasmic reticulum is probably involved (Froelich, Lakatta, & Beard, 1978), together with a lessening of the normal inotropic response to catecholamines.

CONCLUSIONS

We may conclude that, in most people, the decline of maximum oxygen intake with age must be attributed largely to a deterioration of cardiac function rather than to a change of habitual activity or a limitation of effort by some noncardiac factor. The primary influence is a slowing of maximum heart rate. There is also some narrowing of the maximum arterio-venous oxygen difference. Many factors, including a decrease of preloading, an increase of afterloading, and a lesser inotropic action of catecholamines limit the possibility of a compensating increase of stroke volume, despite some left ventricular hypertrophy. While an increase of stroke volume may occasionally develop in special subsamples of the older population, it does not seem a general phenomenon even in those who remain both healthy and physically active. Hence, even the well-trained athlete must accept a 5-6% decrease of aerobic power per decade of adult life.

REFERENCES

ASMUSSEN, E., & Mathiasen, P. (1962). Some physiological functions in physical education students reinvestigated after 25 years. *Journal of the American Geriatric Society*, **10**, 379-387.

ÅSTRAND, P.O. (1986). Exercise physiology of the mature athlete. In J.R. Sutton & R.M. Brock (Eds.), *Sports medicine for the mature athlete* (pp. 3-13). Indianapolis: Benchmark Press.

DEHN, M., & Bruce, R.A. (1972). Longitudinal variations in maximal oxygen intake with age and activity. *Journal of Applied Physiology*, **33**, 805-807.

DEMPSEY, J. (1987). Exercise-induced imperfections in pulmonary gas exchange. *Canadian Journal of Applied Sport Sciences* **12**(Suppl.), 665-705.

FROELICH, J.P., Lakatta, E.G., & Beard, E. (1978). Studies of sarcoplasmic reticulum function and contraction duration in young adult and aged rat myocardium. *Journal of Molecular and Cellular Cardiology*, **10**, 427-438.

GERSTENBLITH, G., Fredericksen, J., Yin, F.C., Fortuin, N.J., Lakatta, E.G., & Weisfeldt, M.L. (1977). Echocardiographic assessment of a normal adult aging population. *Circulation*, **56**, 273-278.

GERSTENBLITH, G., Lakatta, E.G., & Weisfeldt, M.L. (1976). Age changes in myocardial function and exercise response. *Progress in Cardiovascular Diseases*, **19** 1-21.

GIBBONS, L.K., Cooper, K.H., Martin, R.P., & Pollock, M.L. (1977). Medical examination and electrocardiographic analysis of elite distance runners. *Annals of the New York Academy of Sciences,* **301,** 283-296.

GRIMBY, G., Nilsson, N.J., & Saltin, B. (1966). Cardiac output during submaximal and maximal exercise in active middle-aged athletes. *Journal of Applied Physiology,* **21,** 1150-1156.

GRIMBY, G., & Saltin, B. (1966). Physiological analysis of physically well-trained middle-aged and old athletes. *Acta Medica Scandinavica,* **179,** 513-526.

GRIMBY, G., & Saltin, B. (1971). Physiological effects of physical conditioning. *Scandinavian Journal of Rehabilitation Medicine,* **3,** 6-14.

HAGBERG, J.M., Allen, W.K., Seals, D.R., Hurley, B.F., Ehsani, A.A., & Holloszy, J.O. (1985). A hemodynamic comparison of young and older endurance athletes during exercise. *Journal of Applied Physiology,* **58,** 2041-2046.

HANSON, J., Tabakin, B., Levy, A., & Nedde, W. (1968). Long-term physical training and cardiovascular dynamics in middle-aged men. *Circulation,* **38,** 783-789.

HEATH, G.W., Hagberg, J.M., Ehsani, A.A., & Holloszy, J.O. (1981). A physiological comparison of young and older endurance athletes. *Journal of Applied Physiology,* **51,** 634-640.

HODKINSON, H.M., & Pomerance, A. (1977). The clinical significance of senile cardiac amyloidosis: A prospective clinico-pathological study. *Quarterly Journal of Medicine,* **46,** 381-387.

HOLLMANN, W. (1965). *Korperliches Training als Pravention von Herz-Kreislauf Krankheiten.* Stuttgart, W. Germany: Hippokrates Verlag.

JONES, N.L. (1984). Dyspnea in exercise. *Medicine and Science in Sports and Exercise,* **16,** 14-19.

KASCH, F.W., & Kulberg, J. (1981). Physiological variables during 15 years of endurance exercise. *Scandinavian Journal of Sports Science,* **3,** 59-62.

KASCH, F.W., & Wallace, J.P. (1976). Physiological variables during 10 years of endurance exercise. *Medicine and Science in Sports,* **8,** 5-8.

KAVANAGH, T., & Shephard, R.J. (1977). The effects of continued training on the aging process. *Annals of the New York Academy of Sciences,* **301,** 656-670.

KAVANAGH, T., & Shephard, R.J. (in preparation). *Community impact of masters' athleticism on health and aging.*

KAY, C., & Shephard, R.J., (1969). On muscle strength and the threshold of anaerobic work. *Internationale Zeitschrift für Angewandte Physiologie,* **27,** 311-328.

LAKATTA, E.G. (1980). Age-related alterations in cardiovascular response to adrenergic mediated stress. *Federation Proceedings,* **39,** 3173-3177.

LAKATTA, E.G., Mitchell, J.H., Pomerance, A., & Rowe, G.G. (1987). Human aging: Changes in structure and function. *Journal of the American College of Cardiology,* **10,** 42A-47A.

LINZBACH, A.J., & Akuamoa-Boateng, E. (1973). Changes in the aging human heart. I. Heart weight and the aged. *Klinische Wochenschrift,* **51,** 156-163.

MONTOYE, H.J. (1975). *Physical activity and health: An epidemiological study of an entire community.* Englewood Cliffs, NJ: Prentice-Hall.

NIINIMAA, V., & Shephard, R.J. (1978). Training and exercise conductance in the elderly. (2) The cardiovascular system. *Journal of Gerontology, 33,* 362-367.

NISHIMURA, T., Yamada, Y., & Kawai, C. (1980). Echocardiographic evaluation of long-term effects of exercise on left ventricular hypertrophy and function in professional bicyclists. *Circulation, 61,* 832-840.

O'ROURKE, M.F. (1982). *Aging and arterial function* (pp. 185-195). New York: Churchill Livingstone.

PARKER, J.O., diGiorgi, S., & West, R.O. (1966). A haemodynamic study of coronary insufficiency precipitated by exercise. With observations on the effects of nitroglycerine. *American Journal of Medicine, 17,* 470-483.

POLLOCK, M.L., Miller, H.S., Linnerud, A.C., Royster, C.L., Smith, W.E., & Sonner, W.E. (1974). Physiological characteristics of champion American track athletes 40–75 years of age. *Journal of Gerontology, 29,* 645-649.

PORT, S., Cobb, F.R., Coleman, R.E., & Jones, R.H. (1980). Effect of age on the response of the left ventricular ejection fraction to exercise. *New England Journal of Medicine, 303,* 1133-1137.

RAHE, R.H., & Arthur, R.J. (1975). Swim performance decrement over middle life. *Medicine and Science in Sports, 7,* 53-58.

RIEGEL, P.S. (1981). Athletic records and human endurance. *American Scientist, 69,* 285-290.

RODE, A., & Shephard, R.J. (1984). Ten years of "civilization"—Fitness of Canadian Inuit. *Journal of Applied Physiology, Respiratory Environmental and Exercise Physiology, 56,* 1472-1477.

RODEHEFFER, R.J., Gerstenblith, G., Becker, C.C., Fleg, J.L., Weisfeldt, M.L., & Lakatta, E.G. (1984). Exercise cardiac output is maintained with advancing age in healthy human subjects: Cardiac dilatation and increased stroke volume compensation for a diminished heart rate. *Circulation, 69,* 203-213.

SALTIN, B. (1986). Physiological characteristics of the masters athlete. In J.R. Sutton & R.M. Brock (Eds.), *Sports medicine for the mature athlete* (pp. 59-80). Indianapolis: Benchmark Press.

SCHOCKEN, D.D., Blumenthal, J.A., Port, S., Hindle, P., & Coleman, R.E. (1983). Physical conditioning and left ventricular performance in the elderly: Assessment by radionuclide angiocardiography. *American Journal of Cardiology, 52,* 359-364.

SHEPHARD, R.J. (1977). *Endurance fitness* (2nd ed.). Toronto: University of Toronto Press.

SHEPHARD, R.J. (1978). *Human physiological work capacity.* London: Cambridge University Press.

SHEPHARD, R.J. (1987). *Physical activity and aging* (2nd ed.). London: Croom Helm.

SIDNEY, K.H., & Shephard, R.J. (1977a). Maximum and submaximum exercise tests in men and women in the seventh, eighth and ninth decades of life. *Journal of Applied Physiology, 43,* 280-287.

SIDNEY, K.H., & Shephard, R.J. (1977b). Training and E.C.G. abnormalities in the elderly. *British Heart Journal,* **39**, 1114-1120.

SJÖGREN, A.L. (1971). Left ventricular wall thickness in 100 subjects without heart disease. *Chest,* **60**, 341-346.

SPURGEON, H.A., Steinbech, M.F., & Lakatta, E.G. (1983). Chronic exercise prevents characteristic age-related changes in rat cardiac contraction. *American Journal of Physiology,* **244** (Heart, Circulatory Physiology), H513-H518.

STONES, M.J., & Kozma, A. (1980). Adult age trends in athletic performances. *Experimental Aging Research,* **7**, 269-280.

STONES, M.J., & Kozma, A. (1982). Sex differences in changes with age in record running performances. *Canadian Journal on Aging,* **1**, 12-16.

TIPTON, C.M. (1984). Exercise, training and hypertension. *Exercise Sports Science Reviews,* **12**, 245-306.

UNVERFERTH, D.V., Fetters, J.K., & Unverferth, B.J., (1983). Human myocardial histologic characteristics in congestive heart failure. *Circulation,* **68**, 1194-1200.

WEISFELDT, M.L., Gerstenblith, G., & Lakatta, E.G. (1985). Alterations in circulatory function. In R. Andres, E.L. Bierman, & W.R. Hazzard (Eds.), *Principles of geriatric medicine* (pp. 248-279). New York: McGraw-Hill.

Acknowledgment

The gerontological studies of this laboratory are supported in part by a research development grant from the University of Toronto.

Effect of Exercise and Training on Older Men and Women With Essential Hypertension

James M. Hagberg
University of Florida

PREVALENCE OF HYPERTENSION IN OLDER INDIVIDUALS

Of the various diseases that afflict the elderly, hypertension is the most prevalent, the one most closely related to mortality and morbidity, and the one most amenable to treatment (Kannel & Gordon, 1978; Ostfeld, 1986). Most epidemiologic and longitudinal studies have shown that systolic blood pressure at rest increases by approximately 1 mmHg per year from adolescence, while diastolic pressure increases 15–25 mmHg from age 10 to 50 and then remains unchanged (Kaplan, 1986).

However, in Third World countries aging is *not* associated with an increase in either systolic or diastolic blood pressure if the level of acculturation remains the same (Epstein & Eckhoff, 1967; Page & Friedlaender, 1986). In those Third World societies where industrialization, urbanization, and acculturation do occur, the increase in blood pressure with increasing age is of the same magnitude as that in Western societies. Third World populations that do not increase their blood pressure as they age also generally do not show an increase in body weight or fat as they age, unlike persons aging in a Western society. Thus, while the trend in most developed countries in the world is for blood pressure to increase as a person ages, this may be a result of lifestyle changes rather than an immutable and direct concomitant of the normal aging process.

The final result of this increase in blood pressure associated with aging in Western societies is that by age 60, 30–50% of the population has blood pressure in the hypertensive range (Kaplan, 1986; Ostfeld, 1986). This translates into over 20 million people over age 60 in the United States in 1983 afflicted by this disease (Kaplan, 1986). Older individuals also have a type of hypertension that is almost nonexistent in younger populations. Isolated systolic hypertension, defined as a systolic pressure in excess of 160 mmHg and a diastolic pressure below 95 mmHg, is found in less than 1% of the population below the age of 45 but is present in nearly a third of those over 75 years of age (Kaplan, 1986). Isolated systolic hypertension is believed to be the result of decreased arterial elasticity, so that pressure increases to a greater extent during the ejection phase of the cardiac cycle.

HYPERTENSION AS A RISK FACTOR
FOR CARDIOVASCULAR MORTALITY AND MORBIDITY
IN OLDER INDIVIDUALS

Hypertension in young and middle-aged populations is associated with a threefold higher risk for stroke and congestive heart failure, and a twofold higher risk for coronary heart disease and intermittent claudication (Kannel, Doyle, & Ostfeld, 1984). Hypertension persists as a risk factor in populations 60–85 years of age and, in fact, data from the Framingham study indicate that elevated blood pressure in this age group is the *primary* risk factor for cardiovascular mortality and morbidity (Kannel & Gordon, 1978). However, in the very old, those over 85 years of age, the situation seems to be completely reversed; that is, those with the highest blood pressure have a three- to fourfold *lower* mortality than those with lower blood pressure. This finding has been attributed to the fact that those susceptible to the effects of high blood pressure may have already succumbed from its consequences and/or a low blood pressure may be indicative of a disease-related cardiovascular decompensation in the very old (Rajala, Haavisto, Heikinheimo, & Mattila, 1983).

Recent data from clinical trials in Europe (Amery et al., 1985), Australia (Management Committee, 1981), and the United States (Veterans Administration, 1972) indicate that the pharmacologic reduction of blood pressure in older individuals markedly decreases their incidence of cardiovascular diseases. In this regard older populations appear to respond the same as younger groups with essential hypertension (Kaplan, 1986). What is disheartening about the treatment of high blood pressure in older individuals is that many physicians believe that an elevated blood pressure is a normal concomitant of the aging process. This belief has perhaps contributed to the general trend for physicians to be less inclined to prescribe antihypertensive medications for older persons than for younger individuals with the same blood pressure (Kannel & Gordon, 1978). However, the concept that older men and women tolerate this higher pressure better than do younger individuals is not valid. Kannel and Gordon (1978) have clearly shown that the absolute and relative risk associated with a given elevation in blood pressure is increased, not decreased, in older individuals.

EFFECT OF ACUTE EXERCISE ON OLDER INDIVIDUALS
WITH ESSENTIAL HYPERTENSION

Before assessing the potential role that regular physical activity may play in reducing high blood pressure in otherwise healthy older men and women, we must first understand their responses to a single bout of exercise to ensure that they have no contraindications for participating in exercise. This is especially important in older hypertensives because peripheral resistance is higher during exercise in young hypertensives than in their normotensive peers (Amery, Julius, Whitlock, & Conway, 1967; Lund-Johansen, 1967), and peripheral resistance is also higher during exercise in healthy older, compared to younger, men (Hagberg et al., 1985; Julius, Amery, Whitlock, & Conway, 1967). Thus, if the effects of age and hypertension on peripheral resistance during exercise are additive or synergistic, the resultant blood pressure could place an excessive demand on the myocardium to generate the cardiac output necessary at a given submaximal work rate. Also, since even normotensive older men and women have some degree of left ventricular hypertrophy (Henry, Gardin, & Ware, 1980; Sjogren, 1971), if older hypertensives also have an exaggerated blood pressure response to exercise it could markedly increase the demand on their myocardium and place them at a higher risk for a cardiovascular event during exercise.

Studies that have assessed the hemodynamics underlying hypertension in older men and women have generally shown that, compared to most younger hypertensives, older persons have a normal cardiac output with an increased peripheral resistance (Lund-Johansen, 1967; Montain, Jilka, Ehsani, & Hagberg, in press; Terasawa, Kuramoto, Ying, Suzuki, & Kuramochi, 1972). Recently we have shown that this increase in peripheral resistance in older essential hypertensives persists during submaximal exercise at intensities similar to those prescribed in most rehabilitation and fitness programs (Montain et al., in press). This elevated peripheral resistance was accompanied by a cardiac output approximately 10% lower in the hypertensives than in their normotensive peers at the same O_2 consumption. The lower cardiac output in the older hypertensives was the result of a lower stroke volume since both groups had the same heart rate. In addition, the hypertensives had a larger arteriovenous O_2 difference at submaximal work rates to offset their lower cardiac output and arrive at the same O_2 consumption. Therefore, the lower cardiac output in the older hypertensives could potentially reduce the energy demand on their myocardium in the face of the increased resistance to flow in their vascular system. Thus it appears that these individuals may not undergo an excessive myocardial demand during submaximal levels of exercise that would be prescribed in a conventional rehabilitation or fitness exercise program.

In younger hypertensive individuals, a 30- to 45-minute period of moderate-intensity exercise has been shown to reduce systolic blood pressure by as much as 20 mmHg for 1 to 3 hours after exercise, with little or no change in diastolic pressure (cf. Kaufman, Hughson, & Schaman, 1987; Kral, Chrastek, & Adamirova, 1966). We have recently found that this same response is also evident in older men and women with essential hypertension (Hagberg, Montain, & Martin, 1987). Following 45 minutes of exercise at 50% of maximal O_2 consumption ($\dot{V}O_2$max), their systolic blood pressure was reduced by 8 to 12 mmHg for 1 hour compared to those measured at rest prior to exercise. Systolic blood pressure was reduced by 12 to 20 mmHg for 2 hours following 45 minutes of exercise at 70% of $\dot{V}O_2$ max. Diastolic blood pressure was not consistently reduced in either study.

Most previous studies have proposed that this reduction in blood pressure following an acute bout of submaximal exercise is the result of a decrease in peripheral resistance elicited during the exercise that persists during the recovery period (cf. Kaufman et al., 1987). However, our studies of older hypertensives indicate that peripheral resistance returns to baseline resting levels almost immediately after exercise and, if anything, *increases* slightly during the remainder of the recovery period, rather than decreasing (Hagberg et al., 1987). Thus, the reduction in blood pressure following exercise in these older individuals with essential hypertension was the result of a reduction in cardiac output, which in turn was due to a lower stroke volume. Overton, Joyner, and Tipton (1988) have reported somewhat similar findings in spontaneously hypertensive rats. Thus it appears that in individuals with essential hypertension a single session of submaximal exercise can result in reductions in systolic pressure that persist for 1 to 3 hours and, at least in older individuals with hypertension, this reduction in blood pressure appears to be the result of a reduction in cardiac output rather than a vasodilation that persists from the exercise into the recovery period. It is not known if older hypertensives differ from younger hypertensives in the hemodynamics underlying this response following exercise, since cardiac output and peripheral resistance have not been measured in similar studies on younger individuals.

EFFECT OF EXERCISE TRAINING
ON OLDER INDIVIDUALS WITH HYPERTENSION

Until only recently it was believed that men and women over 60 years of age could not elicit an increase in $\dot{V}O_2$ max as a result of endurance exercise training (see Hagberg, 1987), thus inferring that they were incapable of responding to stimuli known to elicit adaptations in younger individuals. However, we have shown that a year-long exercise training program in healthy 60- to 69-year-old men and women increased their $\dot{V}O_2$max by 32% (Seals, Hagberg, Hurley, Ehsani, & Holloszy, 1984a). We have also recently shown that healthy 70- to 78-year-old men and women increased their $\dot{V}O_2$max by an average of 22% with a 6-month endurance exercise training program (Hagberg, Graves, Limacher, et al., 1988). These increases in $\dot{V}O_2$max with prolonged training are in the upper range of what could be expected in younger individuals (Pollock, 1973), leading us to conclude that older healthy men and women are capable of eliciting training adaptations, perhaps within their cardiovascular systems, that result in an increase in $\dot{V}O_2$max.

Only recently has it been concluded that endurance exercise training has a beneficial effect on the blood pressure of younger individuals with essential hypertension (Bjorntorp, 1987; Hagberg, in press). Most early studies investigating the effect of training on hypertensives were flawed by numerous critical design deficiencies (Seals & Hagberg, 1984). They also have generally studied middle-aged individuals. In addition, only Tipton, Matthes, Marcus, Rowlett, and Leininger (1983) have studied older animals with hypertension, reporting that older spontaneously hypertensive rats that were subjected to endurance exercise training exhibited a slower increase in blood pressure than did sedentary age-matched spontaneously hypertensive rats.

Fitness levels have long been known to correlate inversely with blood pressure, though again the majority of these data have been derived from adolescent, young adult, and middle-aged populations (Fraser, Phillips, & Harris, 1983; Kral et al., 1966; Montoye, Metzner, & Keller, 1972). However, recently Heath, Hagberg, Ehsani, and Holloszy (1981) and Pollock, Foster, Knapp, Rod, and Schmidt (1987) found that blood pressure averaged approximately 125/80 mmHg in two groups of highly trained endurance athletes with average ages of 59 and 62 years, respectively, in whom blood pressure would be expected to average 140/85 (Kaplan, 1986). Thus, since it has been shown that older persons can respond to exercise training with adaptations that may involve the cardiovascular system, and since younger hypertensives lower their blood pressure with endurance exercise training, there does appear to be some rationale to infer that exercise training might lower the blood pressure of otherwise healthy older men and women with essential hypertension.

However, the first two studies that assessed the effects of exercise training on older individuals with essential hypertension produced generally negative results. Weber, Barnard, and Roy (1986) reported that exercise training did not lower the blood pressure of 46 men and women, with an average age of 79 years, who had an initial pressure of 154/80 mmHg. Barry and co-workers (1966) found that eight men and women 55–78 years of age, who had an initial blood pressure of 148/88, had a significant decrease in systolic blood pressure on one day of retesting after training but not on a second day of retesting. However, these studies used relatively short training programs lasting only 4 and 13 weeks, respectively.

We recently completed a 9-month study of the effects of exercise training on 60- to 69-year-old men and women with essential hypertension (Hagberg, Montain, Martin, & Ehsani, 1988). This study was designed to determine if low-intensity exercise training was more effective in reducing blood pressure, a possibility raised by the recent findings of Tipton et al. (1983) in spontaneously hypertensive rats. A low-intensity training group trained at an average of 53% of their $\dot{V}O_2$max and a moderate-intensity group trained at an average of 73% of their $\dot{V}O_2$max. The low-intensity group did not increase their $\dot{V}O_2$max as a result of the exercise training program, whereas the moderate-intensity training group increased theirs by an average of 27%. However, the low-intensity training group decreased their systolic blood pressure by 20 mmHg, from 164 to 144. This change was significantly greater than that found in the control group and the moderate-intensity training group. In fact, though the moderate-intensity training group decreased their systolic blood pressure by an average of 8 mmHg, this change was not significantly different from that in the hypertensive control group. Both groups lowered their diastolic blood pressure to the same degree (11–12 mmHg). Thus, despite the lack of change in $\dot{V}O_2$max in the low-intensity exercise training group, they elicited reductions in blood pressure with training that were the same as, or greater than, those elicited by the moderate-intensity training group who had a substantial increase in $\dot{V}O_2$max.

Thus it appears that endurance exercise training in older individuals with essential hypertension can elicit the same reductions in blood pressure as have been shown in younger individuals (Hagberg, in press). This conclusion is also supported by previous meta-analysis results indicating that the magnitude of the reduction in blood pressure elicited by exercise training was not related to the subject's age ($r = -0.13$, and -0.08 for systolic and diastolic pressures, respectively, P=n.s.) (Hagberg, in press).

SUMMARY

Endurance exercise training appears to have the same potential to lower both systolic and diastolic blood pressure in individuals over the age of 60 as it does in younger essential hypertensives. The magnitude of the reduction averages approximately 10 mmHg. From an epidemiological point of view it may be noteworthy that low-intensity training, which would place these older individuals at a much lower cardiovascular and orthopedic risk, appears to lower blood pressure as much or more than higher intensity training.

Reductions in blood pressure of the magnitude found in these older individuals with exercise training have been associated with 20–60% reductions in cardiovascular mortality and morbidity in previous clinical trials assessing the efficacy of antihypertensive medications in the elderly (Amery et al., 1985; Management Committee, 1981). Thus, while exercise training does not appear to completely normalize the blood pressure of most older, otherwise healthy individuals with essential hypertension, the reduction in blood pressure resulting from exercise training does have substantial clinical significance. Therefore it would appear prudent to include exercise training as part of a nonpharmacological approach to the treatment of mild to moderate elevations in blood pressure in the elderly.

This conclusion is also partly based on the fact that while all exercise training studies of these individuals do not demonstrate significant reductions in blood pressure, *no* evidence is available to indicate that such exercise training increases the blood pressure of these individuals. And even if blood pressure is not reduced with endurance exercise training, other risk factors may change favorably to reduce their risk for cardiovascular disease (Seals, Hagberg, Hurley, Ehsani, & Holloszy, 1984b). In addition, even the individual bouts of exercise may produce a transient reduction in systolic blood pressure following exercise.

REFERENCES

AMERY, A., Birkenhäger, W., Brixko, P., Bulpitt, C., Clement, D., Deruytte, M., Deschaep, A., Dollery, C., Fagard, R., & Forette, F. (1985). Mortality and morbidity results from the European Working Party on high blood pressure in the elderly. *Lancet,* **1,** 1349-1355.

AMERY, A., Julius, S., Whitlock, L.S., & Conway, J. (1967). Influence of hypertension on the hemodynamic response to exercise. *Circulation,* **36,** 231-237.

BARRY, A.C., Daly, J.W., Pruett, E.D.R., Steinmetz, J.R., Page, H.F., Birkhead, N.C., & Rohahl, K. (1966). The effects of physical conditioning on older individuals. I. Work capacity, circulatory–respiratory function, and work electrocardiogram. *Journal of Gerontology,* **21,** 182-191.

BJORNTORP, P. (1987). Effects of physical training on blood pressure in hypertension. *European Heart Journal* (Suppl. B), 71-76.

EPSTEIN, F.H., & Eckhoff, R.D. (1967). The epidemiology of high blood pressure— Geographic and etiological factors. In J. Stamler & R. Stamler (Eds.), *The epidemiology of hypertension* (pp. 155-166). New York: Grune & Stratton.

FRASER, G.E., Phillips, R.L., & Harris, R. (1983). Physical fitness and blood pressure in school children. *Circulation,* **67,** 405-412.

HAGBERG, J.M. (1987). Effect of training on the decline of $\dot{V}O_2$ max with aging. *Federation Proceedings,* **46,** 1830-1833.

HAGBERG, J.M. (in press). *Exercise, fitness, and hypertension.* Champaign, IL: Human Kinetics.

HAGBERG, J.M., Allen, W.K., Seals, D.R., Hurley, B.F., Ehsani, A.A., & Holloszy, J.O. (1985). A hemodynamic comparison of young and older endurance athletes during exercise. *Journal of Applied Physiology,* **58,** 2041-2046.

HAGBERG, J.M., Graves, J.E., Limacher, M., Woods, D.R., Cononie, C., Leggett, S., Gruber, J., & Pollock, M.L. (1988). *Cardiovascular response of 70-79 year old men and women to endurance and strength training.* Manuscript submitted for publication.

HAGBERG, J.M., Montain, S.J., & Martin, W.H. (1987). Blood pressure and hemodynamic responses after exercise in older hypertensives. *Journal of Applied Physiology, 63*, 270-276.

HAGBERG, J.M., Montain, S.J., Martin, W.H., & Ehsani, A.A. (1988). *Effect of exercise training on 60-69 year old essential hypertensives.* Manuscript submitted for publication.

HAGBERG, J.M., & Seals, D.R. (1987). Exercise training and hypertension. *Acta Medica Scandinavica* (Suppl. 711), 131-136.

HEATH, G.W., Hagberg, J.M., Ehsani, A.A., & Holloszy, J.O. (1981). A physiological comparison of young and older endurance athletes. *Journal of Applied Physiology, 51*, 534-640.

HENRY, W.L., Gardin, J.M., & Ware, J.H. (1980). Echocardiographic measurements in normal subjects from infancy to old age. *Circulation, 62*, 1054-1061.

JULIUS, S., Amery, A., Whitlock, L.S., & Conway, J. (1967). Influence of age on the hemodynamic response to exercise. *Circulation, 36*, 222-230.

KANNEL, W.B., Doyle, J.T., & Ostfeld, A.M. (1984). Original resources for primary prevention of atherosclerotic diseases. *Circulation, 70*, 157A-168A.

KANNEL, W.B., & Gordon, T. (1978). Evaluation of cardiovascular risk in the elderly: The Framingham Study. *Bulletin of the New York Academy of Medicine, 54*, 573-591.

KAPLAN, N. (1986). *Clinical hypertension* (4th ed.). Baltimore: Williams & Wilkins.

KAUFMAN, F.L., Hughson, R.C., & Schaman, J.P. (1987). Effect of exercise on recovery blood pressure in normotensive and hypertensive subjects. *Medicine and Science in Sports and Exercise, 19*, 17-20.

KRAL, J., Chrastek, J., & Adamirova, J. (1966). The hypotensive effect of physical activity in hypertensive subjects. In W. Raab (Ed.), *Prevention of ischemic heart disease: Principles and practice.* Springfield, IL: C.C Thomas.

LUND-JOHANSEN, P. (1967). Hemodynamics in early essential hypertension. *Acta Medica Scandinavica* (Suppl. 482), 1-105.

MANAGEMENT Committee. (1981). Treatment of mild hypertension in the elderly. *Medical Journal of Australia, 2*, 398-402.

MONTAIN, S.J., Jilka, S.M., Ehsani, A.A., & Hagberg, J.M. (in press). Altered hemodynamics at rest and during exercise in older men and women with essential hypertension. *Hypertension.*

MONTOYE, H.J., Metzner, H.L., & Keller, J.B. (1972). Habitual physical activity and blood pressure. *Medicine and Science in Sports, 4*, 175-181.

OSTFELD, A.M. (1986). Epidemiologic overview. In M.J. Horan, G.M. Steinberg, J.B. Dunbar, & E.C. Hadley (Eds.), *Blood pressure regulation and aging: Proceedings from a symposium* (pp. 3-10). New York: Biomedical Information Corp.

OVERTON, A.M., Joyner, M.J., & Tipton, C.M. (in press). Reduction in blood pressure after acute exercise by hypertensive rats. *Journal of Applied Physiology.*

PAGE, L.B., & Friedlaender, J. (1986). Blood pressure, age, and cultural change: A longitudinal study of Solomon Islands populations. In M.J. Horan, G.M. Steinberg, J.B. Dunbar, & E.C. Hadley (Eds.), *NIH blood pressure regulation and aging: Proceedings from a symposium* (pp. 11-25). New York: Biomedical Information Corp.

POLLOCK, M.L. (1973). The quantification of endurance exercise training programs. In J.H. Wilmore (Ed.), *Exercise and sport sciences reviews* (pp. 155-188). New York: Academic Press.

POLLOCK, M.L., Foster, C., Knapp, D., Rod, J.L., & Schmidt, D.H. (1987). Effect of age and training on aerobic capacity and body composition of master athletes. *Journal of Applied Physiology, 62*, 725-731.

RAJALA, S., Haavisto, M., Heikinheimo, R., & Mattila, K. (1983). Blood pressure and mortality in the very old. *Lancet, II*, 520-521.

SEALS, D.R., & Hagberg, J.M. (1984). The effect of exercise training on human hypertension: A review. *Medicine and Science in Sports and Exercise, 16*, 207-215.

SEALS, D.R., Hagberg, J.M., Hurley, B.F., Ehsani, A.A., & Holloszy, J.O. (1984a). Endurance training in older men and women. I. Cardiovascular response to exercise. *Journal of Applied Physiology, 57*, 1024-1029.

SEALS, D.R., Hagberg, J.M., Hurley, B.F., Ehsani, A.A., & Holloszy, J.O. (1984b). Effects of endurance training on glucose tolerance and plasma lipid levels in older men and women. *Journal of the American Medical Association, 252*, 645-649.

SJOGREN, A.L. (1971). Left ventricular wall thickness determined by ultrasound in 100 subjects without heart disease. *Chest, 60*, 341-346.

TERASAWA, F., Kuramoto, K., Ying, L.H., Suzuki, T., & Kuramochi, M. (1972). The study of the hemodynamics in old hypertensive subjects. *Acta Gerontologica Japan, 56*, 47-55.

TIPTON, C.M., Matthes, R.D., Marcus, K.D., Rowlett, K.A., & Leininger, J.R. (1983). Influences of exercise intensity, age, and medication on resting systolic blood pressure of SHR populations. *Journal of Applied Physiology, 55*, 1305-1310.

VETERANS Administration cooperative study group on antihypertensive agents. (1972). Effects of treatment on morbidity in hypertension. III. Influence of age, diastolic pressure, and prior cardiovascular disease: Further analysis of side effects. *Circulation, 45*, 991-1004.

WEBER, F., Barnard, R.J., & Roy, R. (1986). Effects of a high-complex carbohydrate, low-fat diet and daily exercise on individuals 70 years of age and older. *Journal of Gerontology, 38*, 155-161.

Exercise–Drug Interactions in the Older Adult

Jack H. Wilmore
The University of Texas at Austin

Starting shortly after birth, the body's tissues begin the inevitable process of aging. Likewise, pathological changes that become the precursors of chronic degenerative diseases are evident within the first decade of life. Unfortunately, the manifestations of these diseases are appearing at earlier ages (e.g., hypertension in the preteen years and coronary artery disease in the 20s and 30s!). On the positive side, however, scientists now have a much more complete understanding of disease processes, which is allowing them to develop strategies to prevent the early onset of these diseases and to develop more effective clinical treatments for those who are diagnosed with chronic degenerative disease.

Clinical medicine today, as in years past, depends heavily on the pharmacological approach to treatment whereby major advances have had a significant impact on reducing disease, morbidity, and mortality. As just one example, deaths from stroke, which is the third leading cause of death in the United States, have been reduced by 55% from 1964 to 1984 (Office of Disease Prevention and Health Promotion, 1988). Early identification of those with hypertension and treatment with exercise, diet, and drugs have undoubtedly made major contributions to this remarkable decline in mortality.

This paper will focus on one specific classification of drugs, beta-adrenergic blocking drugs, and their interaction with physical activity, both acute bouts of exercise and chronic endurance training. These are among the most widely prescribed medications, being used in the treatment of hypertension, coronary artery disease, and migraine headache among other health problems.

BETA-ADRENERGIC BLOCKING DRUGS

Beta-adrenergic blocking drugs, first introduced in 1966, have become the most widely used class of drugs for the treatment of cardiovascular diseases (Kaplan, 1983). Clinical trials in postmyocardial infarction (MI) patients treated with β-adrenergic blockers provide overwhelming evidence that long-term β-adrenergic blockade reduces subsequent mortality (Friedewald, 1983; May, 1983). β-blockers are also advocated as an alternative to thiazide-type diuretics as the first step in

Adapted with permission from *The Physician and Sportsmedicine* Series on Cardiac Rehabilitation.

the treatment of hypertension (Joint National Committee, 1984). An estimated prevalence of hypertension and myocardial infarction in the United States of over 60 million cases represents a substantial population eligible for treatment with β-blocker medication (American Heart Association, 1988).

Patients who are treated with β-blockers are likely to be ambulatory and involved to some extent with physical activity of varying intensities. A certain subset of this population will be participating in competitive sports or games, or will be involved in physical training programs (e.g., fitness or rehabilitation programs).

Exercise Testing: The Acute Response to Exercise

At submaximal levels of exercise, for the same absolute rate of work, ß-adrenergic blockade results in an attenuation of heart rate of 15–60 beats/min, the magnitude dependent on dosage and individual response (Wilmore, Freund, et al., 1985). Drugs with intrinsic sympathomimetic activity (ISA) attenuate heart rate to a lesser extent at rest and at lower rates of work, but this ISA property decreases as rates of work approach maximum. β-adrenergic blockers that are selective for β_1 receptors are found predominantly in the heart and have effects on heart rate similar to those that are nonselective, that is, that block both β_1 and β_2 receptors at rates of work up to approximately 90% of maximal capacity. At this point, however, heart rate is attenuated more while on nonselective blocking agents (Anderson et al., 1985). The lower maximal heart rate with nonselective agents has been attributed to their blockade of both β_1 and β_2 receptors. With selective agents the β_2 receptors of the heart can be influenced by circulating catecholamines during the last stages of a maximal exercise test.

Stroke volume is increased in almost direct proportion to the decrease in heart rate with β-blockade, allowing cardiac output to remain unaltered, or only slightly reduced (<10% reduction) at the same rate of work. Oxygen consumption at these submaximal rates of work is either unaffected by β-blockade or reduced slightly (Kalis et al., 1988). In fact, the upward drift observed in submaximal oxygen uptake with prolonged steady-state exercise is not present under conditions of nonselective β-blockade when compared with placebo and selective β-blockade (Kalis et al., 1988). When decreases in cardiac output are observed under β-blockade, it is quite possible that this reduction in cardiac output is a response to a reduced oxygen uptake for that same rate of work. Pulmonary ventilation is generally unaffected or slightly reduced at submaximal rates of work when under β-blockade (Wilmore, Freund, et al., 1985).

Few studies have investigated the consequences of β-adrenergic blockade on moderate to long duration work at intensities that approximate occupational levels (e.g., 1 to 8 hours of work at 25 to 45% of one's capacity). Lundborg et al. (1981) studied carbohydrate and lipid metabolism and the capacity to perform prolonged submaximal physical exercise in six young, healthy subjects treated in a randomized double-blind manner for 2 days with either placebo, propranolol (nonselective), or metroprolol (selective). Subjects performed consecutive 30-minute bouts of exercise with intervening 10-minute rest periods at an intensity previously established to elicit a heart rate response of 130 beats/minute ($\sim 50\%$ of the subjects' maximal oxygen uptake [$\dot{V}O_2$max]). Exercise duration was 152 minutes while on placebo, 117 minutes on metoprolol, and 88 minutes on propranolol. Blood glucose levels decreased under all conditions, but most rapidly under propranolol. Likewise, fatty acid levels were attenuated under propranolol compared to the other two treatment conditions. The investigators concluded that β-andrenoceptor blockade diminishes the capacity for prolonged submaximal work by reducing the availability of substrates to the working muscles.

Similar reductions in submaximal endurance capacity were recently reported by van Baak, Bohm, Arends, van Hooff, and Rahn (1987) in hypertensive patients treated with three different β-blocking agents, propranolol (nonselective), pindolol (nonselective with ISA), and metoprolol (β_1 selective) using an identical exercise protocol. Plasma glucose concentrations were reduced only with propranolol; however, plasma potassium concentrations were significantly increased with all three blocking agents.

Gordon et al. (1985) studied the effect of selective and nonselective β-adrenoceptor blockade on thermoregulation during prolonged exercise in the heat (33° C dry bulb). Eleven healthy adult male subjects performed a 2-hour block-stepping procedure at a work rate of 54 W (approximately 32% of their $\dot{V}O_2$ max) under conditions of placebo, propranolol, and atenolol. Two subjects were unable to complete the exercise task while on propranolol. There were no differences between β-blockers with respect to heart rate attenuation during exercise, or in the rectal and skin temperature increases with exercise. The propranolol conditions elicited a significantly greater sweat rate and an increased postexercise serum K^+.

Freund et al. (1987) investigated thermoregulation during prolonged exercise in the heat (32° C dry bulb) under conditions of placebo, propranolol, and atenolol. Fourteen healthy adult males exercised for 90 minutes on a cycle ergometer at a rate of work equivalent to approximately 40% of their $\dot{V}O_2$ max (unblocked), the absolute rate of work being the same for all three trials. Two subjects were unable to complete the 90-minute ride on propranolol, and two additional subjects had extreme difficulty completing the 90-minute ride while on propranolol. Skin blood flow and mean skin temperature were significantly lower during the propranolol trials compared to those in the atenolol and placebo conditions. Cardiac output was also lower on propranolol, while ratings of perceived exertion were higher.

Of particular interest was the fact that rectal temperature did not differ when the propranolol subjects were compared to the placebo and atenolol subjects. This later finding might be explained by possible differences in rectal versus blood temperature (Gordon, Myburgh, Schwellnus, & van Rensburg, 1987). It appears from these results that the body was attempting to maintain central venous pressure, possibly at the expense of thermoregulation. This may have important implications for those on β-blockers who work for several hours or more in the heat and/or humidity.

With respect to maximal exercise, β-adrenergic blockade has been shown to attenuate maximal oxygen uptake in healthy, highly conditioned subjects with high aerobic capacities (Anderson et al., 1985). The effects appear to be more variable with moderately conditioned subjects, and there appears to be little or no effect in those who are considered average or below average in aerobic or cardiorespiratory endurance capacity (Wilmore, Joyner, Freund, Ewy, & Morton, 1985). In angina patients, there is conclusive evidence that β-adrenergic blockade actually increases tolerance to maximal exercise (Beller et al., 1984).

Those with average or below average aerobic capacity, and even some of those who are moderately trained, are able to compensate for major reductions in their submaximal and maximal heart rate by increasing their stroke volume to maintain cardiac output (Wilmore, Freund, et al., 1985). With highly trained athletes, however, the stroke volume has been maximized by years of training. Although they can continue to increase their stroke volume under conditions of β-adrenergic blockade, they are not able to compensate fully (Anderson et al., 1985; Wilmore, Freund, et al., 1985). Thus, they have a reduction in maximal cardiac output capacity, which leads to a reduction in $\dot{V}O_2$ max of up to 15% or more. Of major importance, highly trained endurance athletes do seem to perform much better on cardioselective, or β_1 selective, drugs. This has been substantiated in several recent studies (Anderson et al., 1985; Joyner, Freund, et al., 1987).

In addition to the reduction in maximal heart rate, β-adrenergic blockade also reduces maximal ventilatory capacity, which could well limit maximal endurance capacity (Anderson et al., 1985; Joyner, Freund, et al., 1987; Joyner, Jilka, et al., 1987; Wilmore, Freund, et al., 1985). Joyner, Jilka, et al. (1987) have recently demonstrated that this is the result of an attenuation in tidal volume with nonselective blockade. Apparently, nonselective blockade inhibits the β_2-mediated bronchodilation that normally occurs with increasing levels of exercise.

The Chronic Adaptations to Exercise Training

Is it possible to attain a training or conditioning response with chronic β-adrenergic blockade when sympathetic drive is attenuated? Early studies using patients with known coronary artery disease demonstrated clearly that a training effect can be obtained while under β-blockade (Horgan & Teo, 1983; Laslett, Paumer, Scott-Baier, & Amsterdam, 1983; Pratt et al., 1981; Vanhees, Fagard, & Amery, 1982). However, these studies were generally not well controlled: There was no randomization of subjects into groups, there was no control over the specific β-blocking drugs used or the dosage of the drug, the endpoints of the exercise tests were generally arbitrary, and the classic marker of training, $\dot{V}O_2$ max, was not directly measured.

The first two studies to address this issue in a systematic manner, using a placebo-controlled and a double-blinded design, reported conflicting results. Sable et al. (1982) reported no improvement in $\dot{V}O_2$ max with a 5-week intensive aerobic exercise training program in young, healthy, sedentary men on propranolol, while the control group improved their $\dot{V}O_2$ max by 20.9%. Ewy et al. (1983), using a similar experimental design and drug (sotolol) but a 14-week training program, reported an increase in $\dot{V}O_2$ max with training in their β-blocked group of 6.7%. Their placebo group increased their $\dot{V}O_2$ max by 8.6%. The reason for the disparity in results is not immediately obvious. Subjects in the Sable study trained for only 5 weeks and their training was conducted at altitude (University of Colorado, Denver). However, their control group did demonstrate a substantial training response. Subsequent studies from the University of Colorado group have confirmed their earlier findings, reporting either no training effect (Hiatt, Marsh, Brammell, Fee, & Horwitz, 1984; Marsh, Hiatt, Brammell, & Horwitz, 1983) or an attenuated training effect (Wolfel et al., 1986), using $\dot{V}O_2$ max as the marker of training.

Additional studies of both normal, healthy subjects (McLeod, Kraus, & Williams, 1984; Savin et al., 1985; Wilmore, Ewy, et al., 1985) and patients with coronary artery disease (Ciske, Dressendorfer, Gordon, & Timmis, 1986; McAllister & Lee, 1986; Stuart, Koyal, Lundstrom, Thomas, & Ellestad, 1985) have demonstrated substantial training effects while medicated with β-blockers. Thus, with the exception of the studies from the University of Colorado, it appears that a normal training effect can be achieved while under the influence of β-adrenergic blockade in both normal, healthy individuals as well as in patients with coronary artery disease.

β-Adrenergic Blockade: Implications for Exercise Prescription

The results of those studies cited in the previous sections of this paper have important implications for the prescription of exercise in patients who have been prescribed β-adrenergic blocking agents. First, these patients should have their exercise prescription based on the results of treadmill or cycle ergometer testing conducted while medicated. The derivation of a training heart rate range must be based on an exercise test conducted under conditions as similar as possible, with respect to the timing of medication, to those under which the individual will be exercising. For example, maximal heart rate at the time of the peak response to medication may be 140 beats/min or lower. However, with a short-acting agent the maximal heart rate 4–6 hours after the peak response will be considerably higher. While a training heart rate range of 105 to 120 beats/min would be adequate at the time of peak response, it would be considerably below the training threshold at 4 to 6 hours after the peak response (Wilmore, Freund, et al., 1985).

Second, it is appropriate to consider the use of cardioselective agents, since they appear to present more favorable conditions under which to exercise with respect to their effects on endurance capacity, ventilation, thermoregulation, and trainability (Wilmore, Freund, et al., 1985). Finally, there appears to be no problem in training individuals who are taking β-blockers, providing they follow the standard guidelines for exercise prescription as outlined by the American College of Sports Medicine (1986).

REFERENCES

AMERICAN College of Sports Medicine. (1986). *Guidelines for exercise testing and prescription* (3rd ed.). Philadelphia: Lea & Febiger.

AMERICAN Heart Association. (1988). *Heart Facts 1988*. Dallas: Author.

ANDERSON, R.L., Wilmore, J.H., Joyner, M.J., Freund, B.J., Hartzell, A.A., Todd, C.A., & Ewy, G.A. (1985). Effects of cardio-selective and nonselective beta-adrenergic blockade on the performance of highly trained runners. *American Journal of Cardiology,* **55**, 149D-154D.

BELLER, G.A., Bittar, N., Coelho, J.B., Craddock, G.B., Ezekowitz, M.D., Murray, G.C., Steen, S.N., & Waksman, J.A. (1984). Double-blind, placebo-controlled trial of propranolol given once, twice and four times daily in stable angina pectoris: A multicenter study using serial exercise testing. *American Journal of Cardiology,* **54**, 37-42.

CISKE, P.E., Dressendorfer, R.H., Gordon, S., & Timmis, G.C. (1986). Attenuation of exercise training effects in patients taking beta blockers during early cardiac rehabilitation. *American Heart Journal,* **112**, 1016-1025.

EWY, G.A., Wilmore, J.H., Morton, A.R., Stanforth, P.R., Constable, S.H., Buono, M.J., Conrad, K.A., Miller, H., & Gatewood, C.F. (1983). The effect of beta-adrenergic blockade on obtaining a trained exercise state. *Journal of Cardiac Rehabilitation, 3*, 25-29.

FREUND, B.J., Joyner, M.J., Jilka, S.M., Kalis, J., Nittolo, J.M., Taylor, J.A., Peters, H., Feese, G., & Wilmore, J.H. (1987). Thermoregulation during prolonged exercise in heat: Alterations with beta-adrenergic blockade. *Journal of Applied Physiology, 63*, 930-936.

FRIEDEWALD, W.T. (1983). Beta-adrenergic blockade after myocardial infarction: Clinical and public health implications of the reported beta-blocker clinical trials. *Circulation, 67* (suppl. I), I110-I111.

GORDON, N.F., Kruger, P.E., van Rensburg, J.P., Van Der Linde, A., Kielblock, A.J., & Cilliers, J.F. (1985). Effect of β-adrenoceptor blockade on thermoregulation during prolonged exercise. *Journal of Applied Physiology, 58*, 899-906.

GORDON, N.F., Myburgh, D.P., Schwellnus, M.P., & van Rensburg, J.P. (1987). Effect of β-blockade on exercise core temperature in coronary artery disease patients. *Medicine and Science in Sports and Exercise, 19*, 591-596.

HIATT, W.R., Marsh, R.C., Brammell, H.L., Fee, C., & Horwitz, L.D. (1984). Effect of aerobic conditioning on the peripheral circulation during chronic beta-adrenergic blockade. *Journal of the American College of Cardiology, 4*, 958-963.

HORGAN, J.H., & Teo, K.K. (1983). Training response in patients with coronary artery disease receiving beta-adrenergic blocking drugs with or without partial agonist activity. *Journal of Cardiovascular Pharmacology, 5*, 1019-1024.

JOINT National Committee on Detection, Evaluation, and Treatment of High Blood Pressure: 1984 Report. (1984). *Archives of Internal Medicine, 144*, 1045-1057.

JOYNER, M.J., Freund, B.J., Jilka, S.M., Hetrick, G.A., Martinez, E., Ewy, G.A., & Wilmore, J.H. (1987). Effects of β-blockade on exercise capacity of trained and untrained men: A hemodynamic comparison. *Journal of Applied Physiology, 60*, 1429-1434.

JOYNER, M.J., Jilka, S.M., Taylor, J.A., Kalis, J.K., Nittolo, J., Hicks, R.W., Lohman, T.G., & Wilmore, J.H. (1987). β-blockade reduces tidal volume during heavy exercise in trained and untrained men. *Journal of Applied Physiology, 62*, 1819-1825.

KALIS, J., Freund, B.J., Joyner, M.J., Jilka, S.M., Nittolo, J., & Wilmore, J.H. (1988). Effect of β-blockade on the drift in O_2 consumption during prolonged exercise. *Journal of Applied Physiology, 64*, 753-758.

KAPLAN, N.M. (1983). The present and future use of β-blockers. *Drugs, 25* (Suppl. 2), 1-4.

LASLETT, L.J., Paumer, L., Scott-Baier, P., & Amsterdam, E.A. (1983). Efficacy of exercise training in patients with coronary artery disease who are taking propranolol. *Circulation, 68*, 1029-1034.

LUNDBORG, P., Astrom, H., Bengtsson, C., Fellenius, E., von Schenck, H., Svensson, L., & Smith, U. (1981). Effect of B-adrenoceptor blockade on exercise performance and metabolism. *Clinical Science, 61*, 299-305.

MARSH, R.C., Hiatt, W.R., Brammell, H.L., & Horwitz, L.D. (1983). Attenuation of exercise conditioning by low dose beta-adrenergic receptor blockade. *Journal of the American College of Cardiology, 2*, 551-556.

MAY, G.S. (1983). A review of long-term beta-blocker trials in survivors of myocardial infarction. *Circulation,* **67** (suppl. I), I46-I49.

McALLISTER, R.M., & Lee, S.J.K. (1986). The effects of exercise training in patients with coronary artery disease taking beta blockers. *Journal of Cardiopulmonary Rehabilitation,* **6,** 245-250.

McLEOD, A.A., Kraus, W.E., & Williams, R.S. (1984). Effects of $beta_1$-selective and nonselective beta-adrenoceptor blockade during exercise conditioning in healthy adults. *American Journal of Cardiology,* **53,** 1656-1661.

OFFICE of Disease Prevention and Health Promotion, U.S. Public Health Service. (1988). *Disease prevention/health promotion: The facts.* Palo Alto, CA: Bull Publishing.

PRATT, C.M., Welton, D.E., Squires, W.G., Kirby, T.E., Hartung, G.H., & Miller, R.R. (1981). Demonstration of training effect during chronic beta-adrenergic blockade in patients with coronary artery disease. *Circulation,* **64,** 1125-1129.

SABLE, D.L., Brammell, H.L., Sheehan, M.W., Nies, A.S., Gerber, J., & Horwitz, L.D. (1982). Attenuation of exercise conditioning by beta-adrenergic blockade. *Circulatio,* **65,** 679-684.

SAVIN, W.M., Gordon, E.P., Kaplan, S.M., Hewitt, B.F., Harrison, D.C., & Haskell, W.L. (1985). Exercise training during long-term beta-blockade treatment in healthy subjects. *American Journal of Cardiology,* **55,** 101D-109D.

STUART, R.J., Koyal, S.N., Lundstrom, R., Thomas, L., & Ellestad, M.H. (1985). Does exercise training alter maximal oxygen uptake in coronary artery disease during long-term beta-adrenergic blockade? *Journal of Cardiopulmonary Rehabilitation,* **5,** 410-414.

Van BAAK, M.A., Bohm, R.O.B., Arends, B.G., van Hooff, M.E.J., & Rahn, K.H. (1987). Long-term antihypertensive therapy with beta-blockers: Submaximal exercise capacity and metabolic effects during exercise. *International Journal of Sports Medicine,* **8,** 342-347.

VANHEES, L., Fagard, R., & Amery, A. (1982). Influence of beta adrenergic blockade on effects of physical training in patients with ischemic heart disease. *British Heart Journal,* **48,** 33-38.

WILMORE, J.H., Ewy, G.A., Freund, B.J., Hartzell, A.A., Jilka, S.M., Joyner, M.J., Todd, C.A., Kinzer, S.M., & Pepin, E.B. (1985). Cardiorespiratory alterations consequent to endurance exercise training during chronic beta-adrenergic blockade with atenolol and propranolol. *American Journal of Cardiology,* **55,** 142D-148D.

WILMORE, J.H., Freund, B.J., Joyner, M.J., Hetrick, G.A., Hartzell, A.A., Strother, R.T., Ewy, G.A., & Faris, W.E. (1985). Acute response to submaximal and maximal exercise consequent to beta-adrenergic blockade: Implications for the prescription of exercise. *American Journal of Cardiology,* **55,** 135D-141D.

WILMORE, J.H., Joyner, M.J., Freund, B.J., Ewy, G.A., & Morton, A.R. (1985). Beta-blockade and response to exercise: Influence of training. *Physician and Sportsmedicine,* **13**(7), 60-69.

WOLFEL, E.E., Hiatt, W.R., Brammell, H.L., Carry, M.R., Ringel, S.P., Travis, V., & Horwitz, L.D. (1986). Effects of selective and nonselective $beta$-adrenergic blockade on mechanisms of exercise conditioning. *Circulation,* **74,** 664-674.

PRESIDENTS

American Academy of Physical Education

*1926-30	Clark W. Hetherington	1965-66	Leonard A. Larson
*1930-38	Robert Tait McKenzie	*1966-67	Arthur A. Esslinger
*1938-39	Robert Tait McKenzie	1967-68	Margaret G. Fox
	Mabel Lee	*1968-69	Laura J. Huelster
*1939-41	John Brown, Jr.	1969-70	H. Harrison Clarke
*1941-43	Mabel Lee	1970-71	Ruth M. Wilson
*1943-45	Arthur H. Steinhaus	1971-72	Ben W. Miller
*1945-47	Jay B. Nash	1972-73	Raymond A. Weiss
*1947-49	Charles H. McCloy	1973-74	Ann E. Jewett
*1949-50	Frederick W. Cozens	1974-75	King J. McCristal
*1950-51	Rosalind Cassidy	*1975-76	Leona Holbrook
1951-52	Seward C. Staley	1976-77	Marvin H. Eyler
*1952-53	David K. Brace	1977-78	Louis E. Alley
1953-54	Neils P. Neilson	1978-79	Marguerite A. Clifton
*1954-55	Elmer D. Mitchell	1979-80	Harold M. Barrow
1955-56	Anna S. Espenschade	1980-81	Aileene S. Lockhart
*1956-57	Harry A. Scott	1981-82	Earle F. Zeigler
*1957-58	Charles C. Cowell	1982-83	Edward J. Shea
*1958-59	Delbert Oberteuffer	1983-84	Henry J. Montoye
*1959-60	Helen Manley	1984-85	David H. Clarke
1960-61	Thomas E. McDonough, Sr.	1985-86	G. Alan Stull
1961-62	M. Gladys Scott	1986-87	Margaret J. Safrit
1962-63	Fred V. Hein	1987-88	Robert M. Malina (current)
1963-64	Carl L. Nordly	1987-88	Waneen W. Spirduso (elect)
*1964-65	Eleanor Metheny		

---

*Deceased

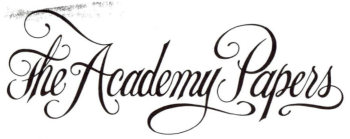

The Academy Papers

With comprehensive coverage of current topics of interest and contributions from the foremost scholars in the field, The Academy Papers are an invaluable resource for every physical education professional and student.

Physical Activity in Early and Modern Populations, Volume 21,
Robert M. Malina, PhD, and Helen M. Eckert, PhD, Editors

The ten papers in this volume detail the evolution of physical activity in society including: early man, modern man's ability to adapt to sedentary occupations, diseases of the advanced society, the health of children, and the health of the aging.
1988 • Paper • 120 pp • Item BMAL0180 • ISBN 0-87322-180-X

The Cutting Edge of Physical Education Research, Volume 20,
Margaret J. Safrit, PhD, and Helen M. Eckert, PhD, Editors

The contributors in this fascinating volume explore the state-of-the-art and the future of research in exercise science, sport and exercise psychology, motor learning, pedagogy, sport history, philosophy of sport, and biomechanics.
1987 • Paper • 136 pp • Item BSAF0098 • ISBN 0-87322-098-6

Effects of Physical Activity on Children, Volume 19,
G. Alan Stull, EdD, and Helen M. Eckert, PhD, Editors

This authoritative volume provides an up-to-date examination of the impact of exercise on the physical, moral, emotional, and intellectual development of children.
1986 • Paper • 174 pp • Item BSTU0049 • ISBN 0-87322-049-8

Limits of Human Performance, Volume 18,
David H. Clarke, PhD, and Helen M. Eckert, PhD, Editors

These intriguing papers explore how age, psychological influences, morphological and physiological characteristics, heat, biomechanics, and other factors can limit performance.
1985 • Paper • 144 pp • Item BCLA0099 • ISBN 0-931250-99-4

Exercise and Health, Volume 17,
Helen M. Eckert, PhD, and Henry J. Montoye, PhD, Editors

Leading scholars provide an extensive analysis of the relationship between exercise and heart disease, osteoporosis, amenorrhea, obesity, aging, arthritis, mental health, and other factors.
1984 • Paper • 160 pp • Item BECK0056 • ISBN 0-931250-56-0

Human Kinetics Publishers, Inc.
Department 265 • Box 5076 • Champaign, IL 61820

Call TOLL FREE for Credit Card Orders
1-800-DIAL-HKP (1-800-342-5457)
1-800-334-3665 (*in Illinois*)
FAX (217) 351-2674
(VISA, AMEX, MC)